The Million Dollar Smile
Changing Lives with Cosmetic Dentistry

The Million Dollar Smile

Changing Lives with Cosmetic Dentistry

Blue Ocean Publishing Group

Dunedin, FL

The Million Dollar Smile
Changing Lives with Cosmetic Dentistry

Published by Blue Ocean Publishing Group
1497 Main St., Ste 236
Dunedin, FL 34698

The information provided within this book is the author's personal thoughts and experience at the time of publishing. While we try to keep the information up-to-date and correct, there are no representations or warranties, express or implied, about the completeness, accuracy, reliability, suitability or availability with respect to the information, products, services, or related graphics contained in this book for any purpose.

There are no income claims or promised results as the application of the ideas and methods described can vary from one person to another.

For permissions contact:
barak@metrixpromotions.com

ISBN: 978-1-947436-01-5

Dedication

*This book is dedicated to you, the reader,
because by picking up this book,
you show you care about your oral health.*

Table of Contents

INTRODUCTION

T his book discusses the benefits of cosmetic dentistry and so much more. It is a resource for you, the patient and the consumer, so that you can learn more about various cosmetic procedures and what they will do for your overall health and well-being. *The Million Dollar Smile: Changing Lives with Cosmetic Dentistry* will help you understand the complex world of cosmetic dentistry so that you can make informed decisions about your oral treatments.

As a dental patient, you have the right to know what procedures are best for you; the risks and benefits of any dental procedure; the cost of all procedures and if insurance will cover part or all of the expense; and what type of outcome you can reasonably expect from the procedure. Unfortunately, many patients are hesitant to ask questions and even worse, are subjected to high-pressure sales pitches designed only to sell expensive dental work by the doctors they should be able to trust.

This book was created to help you understand all the options you have when faced with choices about your oral care. The experts that have contributed to this book have done so because they want patients to understand these procedures. They also want to allow them to make the right decisions about their own healthcare.

Cosmetic dentistry is not a new practice. Archaeological evidence shows that as early as 700 B.C., dentures were made from ivory and bone. Since then, technological advances through the centuries have increased the popularity of cosmetic dental procedures. Certainly, people throughout the ages have recognized the importance of strong teeth; many cultures have also placed a premium on a beautiful smile. The significance of a healthy, attractive smile has never been more important than it is in today's culture. Because of new technology, particularly made possible by the use of computers, you can have the smile of your dreams, provided that you know which procedures will give you the best outcome.

Today, patients are faced with a vast array of cosmetic dental procedures. In fact, there are so many dental procedures available now that it may be overwhelming to consider all the options. Dentists offer services such as:

- Smile Makeovers
- Crowns
- Teeth Whitening
- Periodontal Treatment
- Veneers
- Dentures
- Bridges
- Implants
- Orthodontics
- Treating incorrect bite

Patients of any age, from the very old to the very young, can safely receive most dental treatments. There is even sedation dentistry for those who suffer from extreme anxiety about dental procedures or for those who simply want a more comfortable experience.

In *The Million Dollar Smile: Changing Lives with Cosmetic Dentistry*, 12 leading dentists from around the country educate you, the reader, about subjects related to cosmetic dentistry. Each of these experts is recognized as a successful leader in their various fields. In this book, you will have access to their knowledge and insight on the following topics:

The Importance of a Healthy Attractive Smile – Donald Vespa, DDS, offers insight into how important it really is to have a beautiful smile (hint: it may be more important than you think!)

Today's Crowns are Incognito – Erick V. Pagan, DMD, discusses the importance of crowns and fillings in today's cosmetic dentistry landscape

Fifty Shades of White – Wayne Sutton, DDS, discusses the problem of dull, yellow teeth and how to correct it

The Foundation of a Great Smile – Jessica Stilley, DMD, MS, explains why gum health is the key to overall oral health

Smile Makeover with Porcelain Veneers – Todd Goldstein, DDS, talks about dental veneers and how they can give instant results in brightening and straightening a smile

Biting Right is Living Right – Michael Firouzian, DDS, helps you understand why your bite is so critical to your overall health and how to make it perfect so you can enjoy years of healthy teeth and gums

Straight Talk on Orthodontics – Rita Y. Chuang, DDS, explains the facts regarding braces, including both traditional and Invisalign® methods

Consequences of Missing Teeth – Bruce Seidner, DDS, discusses the health concerns regarding missing teeth and how this problem can be solved

Filling the Gaps with Dental Implants – Jim Eggleston, DDS, helps you understand how dental implants work and whether they are a good choice for you

Leading the Way with Digital Dentistry – Curtis Hayes, DDS, goes over the new technology advances in dentistry that help achieve better and safer results.

No Fear with Sedation Dentistry – J. Derek Tieken, DDS, offers honest opinions on sedation dentistry and its benefits.

Affordable Cosmetic Dentistry Options – Terri Alani, DDS, covers ways you can improve your smile even if you are on a financial stretch and which services will get you the best results on limited funds.

Finally, feel free to jump from one section to another in the book; you do not have to read the chapters in order. Pick your favorite topic and start learning immediately about the things you need to know to make great decisions about your dental care!

The Million Dollar Smile: Changing Lives with Cosmetic Dentistry is your guide to making the right choices for your own oral health. Let our experts help you make the right decisions about your dental care!

THE IMPORTANCE OF A HEALTHY ATTRACTIVE SMILE

Having a great smile is important for a number of reasons. Having – or not having – a great smile affects a person's health, how they're perceived by others, and inevitably how they feel about themselves.

THE IMPACT OF YOUR SMILE

Meeting new people is a daily occurrence in most of our lives. Think back to your last interaction, what was the first thing you did? Did you smile and say hello? Your smile is often one of the first things people notice. If you're not afraid to smile, if you're confident about the look of your smile, others notice. If you consider how you view others, think about what a person's smile usually conveys to you. In most cases, we perceive individuals with great smiles as people that are healthy, attractive, successful, and happy, or at least, not sad, depressed, or disagreeable. When you're out among people, whether you know them well or not, failing to smile- for whatever reason- often conveys a sense of sadness, grumpiness, displeasure, or even anger.

The reasons for people not smiling will vary. It might be because their teeth are less than ideally straight. Perhaps they have fractured, damaged, or stained teeth, or they might be missing teeth. For individuals that suffer from these issues, aesthetics is a major problem. Individuals who suffer from temporomandibular joint problems – TMJ Disorder – or other structural issues with the jaw and mouth may fail to smile because it causes pain or because they're in pain and aren't motivated to smile. Whatever the reason, it's very noticeable when a person consistently fails to smile, and it can and usually does have a significant impact on both their personal and social lives.

SOCIAL CONSEQUENCES

In terms of social exposure, as I mentioned above, having a great smile is important. Successful, happy, healthy people – especially when it comes to those who are constantly exposed to social situations, such as celebrities – have great smiles that they show off all the time. When such individuals, or really anyone with constant social exposure, fail to smile it can be perceived not only as sadness, anger, or pain but also as a cover-up. Failure to smile can signal the inclination or need to hide imperfections or to simply hide anything. It can be an indication that the individual has something to hide. In short, failing to smile conveys a lack of openness, and that can have a significantly negative impact on a person's social life and relationships with others.

In the last few decades, the tools and techniques developed to help people get the perfect smile have increased dramatically. If you take a look at older movies, older celebrities, or even older family photos, smiles weren't as "perfect" decades ago as they tend to be now. With advancements in orthodontics, surgeries, teeth whitening, and other cosmetic procedures – including the major strides made with veneers – the perfect smile gets straighter and whiter all the time. Not everyone has the exact same idea when it comes to a perfect smile but it's safe to say that, as the years have progressed, what is considered a great smile has changed with improvements in dentistry and the tools available to correct and fix a person's smile.

Unfortunately, that also means that the less straight and less white your smile, the more it stands out as being less than what's considered a perfect or great smile. People are aware of this fact, and that leads them to smile in an attempt to cover up imperfections, which then affects how they are perceived by others and ultimately how they feel about themselves.

THE STATISTICS OF APPEARANCE

While it's impossible to provide direct, accurate statistics when it comes to appearance and success, it's fairly easy to notice that many of the world's most successful individuals also tend to be attractive. A great smile is just one part of appearance, which means that it's even more difficult to provide direct, accurate statistics that show individuals with a great smile are substantially more successful than those who lack a great smile or who habitually fail to smile.

That being said, an interesting book by University of Texas' Daniel Hamermesh – entitled *Beauty Pays: Why Attractive People Are More Successful* – provides pages of numbers and data that seem to indicate a direct correlation between success and beauty. The broad point of this book is that attractive people experience advantages when it comes to jobs, opportunities, earnings, and even personal and professional happiness and fulfillment. At the end of the day, this doesn't boil down to a simple equation: a great smile equals success. What it does offer, though, is an idea that most people probably already think is true: how you look – which includes having a nice smile – has a direct impact on your overall success in life.

THE ISSUE OF CONFIDENCE

As I've already mentioned, how you feel about your smile plays a major role in how you feel about yourself. A beautiful smile can leave others with a good first impression of you, whether it's during a job interview, meeting a loved one's family for the first time, or meeting anyone for the first time. A good smile boosts self-confidence. On the other hand, not having a healthy, beautiful smile, one that you're happy to show off, can lead to a substantial lack of confidence, which ultimately affects how you behave and how you feel.

Failing to smile or having a misaligned, stained, broken smile often affects how old a person looks. Along with structural problems, this premature aging of a person's face inevitably affects their confidence and, again, often leads to concealing one's smile.

I've seen this problem frequently in my own practice. It makes perfect sense that a person who isn't confident in their smile doesn't want to smile. They don't want other people to see the issues they have with their teeth, and if and when they do smile, it can be pretty apparent that they're doing their best to conceal the way their smile looks. This, over and over, reflects a lack of self-confidence and self-esteem. It also affects how confident others feel about the individual. Again and again, the issue of confidence has a major impact on a person, often in nearly every arena of their lives. As a dentist, I see this often and it's one of the primary reasons I work so hard to give my patients the best possible treatment and overall care. By offering patients the opportunity to improve their smile, in at least some way I'm also helping them improve their confidence.

THE REALTOR TURNED FLIGHT ATTENDANT

I'd like to share the story of one patient I worked on. Her story, I think, reflects a good deal about how having a great smile affects confidence and success.

This patient – a lady somewhere in her 50s – came to my practice with teeth that were crowded and yellowing. She'd been a realtor for the majority of her professional life and was preparing to follow her dream of switching careers and becoming a flight attendant. She was concerned about the appearance of her smile and how it would affect her in a new professional arena. Clearly, as a flight attendant – especially a brand new flight attendant – having a great smile is super important. Going back to a school environment, being around new people, and starting a new career, she really wanted a beautiful smile.

As I mentioned, her teeth were crowded, they were misaligned, some of her front teeth had chips and fractures, and were stained yellow. I saw her as a patient for several months, trying to work up the best treatment plan and give her the smile she was looking for. We ended up doing eight veneers for her.

She ended up moving out of the area to pursue the new career, but I was able to keep in touch with her for a while. I received a nice note from her when she got into flight school and also when she got a job as a flight attendant. She intimated that having the smile she wanted gave her the confidence to go out and chase her dreams. Taking on a brand-new career in mid-life is an intimidating and challenging undertaking, all the more so if you're not confident in your appearance, which often translates into how confidently you perform in your daily life. Giving her a great smile helped give her the boost she needed to accomplish her goals. Having a great smile isn't everything but it goes a long way towards giving patients the lift they need to challenge themselves and excel in life.

ORAL HEALTH AND TOTAL HEALTH

The importance of a great smile is not only about aesthetics. There are significant practical health considerations as well. Your oral health, in turn, affects your total health. I'd like to offer some data that reflects the general state of American's oral health and how this can have dire consequences for not only a person's smile but for their entire body.

According to the American Dental Hygiene Association (ADHA), 75% of Americans suffer from at least one form of gum disease and are completely unaware of it. In terms of cosmetic dentistry and care for oral health, the American Academy of Cosmetic Dentistry estimates that more patients are female – around 56% – while only about 33% of patients are male. These numbers indicate that having a beautiful, healthy smile is more important to women, although more and more men are coming to have their smiles overhauled. The Gallup Health Race Poll indicated that in the last year – 2016 to 2017 – 34% of the American population didn't visit a dentist at all. This figure is of significant importance to me as a dentist, especially when you remember that three out of four people are suffering from gum issues and don't even know they have a problem.

Visiting a dentist regularly is vital, not only to the beauty of your smile and your oral health but to your health as a whole. The figure related by the ADHA is of particular concern because people with gum disease are more susceptible to suffer from other significant health complications. Individuals with gum disease are almost twice as likely to suffer from coronary artery disease when compared to individuals with no gum disease. On top of this, research has shown that patients with poor oral health care and gum issues also have an increased risk of dementia. Other research shows direct correlations between poor oral health care and blood sugar control, which spikes the number of individuals who suffer from diabetes.

There are a number of other links that can be drawn between oral health and overall health. The studies and research are extensive. While I could fill an entire book up with information about such links, I think it's important to at least list some of the other major health concerns that stem from – or are directly linked to – poor oral hygiene and gum disease. These concerns include breathing problems, respiratory infections, and fertility issues.

The bottom line is this: we need to encourage patients to visit a dentist regularly, regardless of whether they think they have any problems, aesthetic or otherwise. When three out of every four Americans are walking around with gum disease, unaware, coupled with the links to other major health complications, that's a serious problem.

SPECIFIC MOUTH AND JAW ISSUES

Dental problems tend to result in a chain reaction that leads to ever greater and more serious problems. Poor oral hygiene leads to periodontal disease – gum disease – which then leads to a deterioration of the gums, which then affects the structure of the entire mouth. Gum recession and tooth loss lead to structural breakdowns where bone loss occurs, and that leads to more teeth becoming loose and eventually being lost. Down the road, this can lead to a full loss of teeth and people getting dentures. However, getting plastic teeth, while one option of replacement, isn't a sufficient treatment for bone loss and structural breakdowns.

It's also important to remember that these issues are often coupled with the other overall health concerns I mentioned previously.

The goal then needs to be preventing gum disease before it happens with proper oral hygiene and regular dentist visits. These visits are critical because they offer patients a professional, complete cleaning that can't be accomplished at home, and because a dentist can easily spot problems long before they become apparent to patients. These visits also help patients learn about any oral health concerns that may have arisen and make it easier to stop the progression of problem issues early on before they cause major damage that is much more difficult – and expensive – to repair.

One major oral health concern that I feel needs to be mentioned specifically is oral cancer. While a regular dentist can't specifically diagnose and treat oral cancer, they are attuned to signs and symptoms indicating it might be a concern. I do screens for oral cancer in all of my patients. The goal is to catch it before it happens or to stop it before it spreads.

The primary point is this: going to the dentist is not just about checking for simple decay. We check for many things that you might not see or notice. The goal is prevention and early detection. Seeing a dentist regularly increases your chances of catching issues before they become full-blown disease and make it dramatically easier to prevent problems from getting further out of hand. Diagnosing and treating any issue, particularly when it comes to the mouth, should be done immediately. Seeing your dentist regularly makes this possible. I see patients every day who have lost some or all of their natural teeth and simply wish they could have them back. It's far easier and less costly to maintain your oral health than it is to correct serious problems once the damage to mouth has been done.

COMMON SMILE PROBLEMS

There are a variety of reasons why an individual might not be happy or satisfied with their smile. One of the most common cosmetic issues I see with patients is teeth discoloration. If this is a result of decay, then of course more than purely cosmetic treatment is needed. However, a lot of people see greater and greater discoloration due to the things they eat and drink. Coffee, tea, and wine are all harsh on teeth. Because of this, dentists are seeing more patients who are seeking bleaching or some type of whitening treatment.

Another common problem is crooked and misaligned teeth. This can be caused by a number of things, but orthodontics is usually a good way to fix such problems. If these issues are a result of gum disease, then the gum issues need to be addressed.

In most of my patients' cases, they come to me and tell me something specific about their smile that makes them unhappy. Discoloration, crowded or crooked teeth, missing teeth – all of these things can be addressed from a cosmetic standpoint. However, dentists do have to look at the overall health and structure of their mouth and jaw to determine what full course of treatment needs to be pursued because while cosmetic adjustments are highly desired, they are not always the only issue that needs to be corrected.

In terms of treatment that patients seem to request more and more these days, many come in looking for veneers. Veneers are a great solution for a number of cosmetic issues, including discoloration, crooked and missing teeth, and even crowding in some situations. I started doing veneers for patients in the 1980s when they were first introduced. They've come a long way over the past 30 years and often give my patients the smile they're looking for.

EDUCATION AND TRAINING OF DENTISTS

Whatever type of treatment you're receiving, it's always important to look for doctors, dentists, and surgeons with education, training, and experience. What's particularly sad to realize, at least for me, is that a number of people offer cosmetic dentistry treatment without necessarily having the proper education and experience to back it up. The ADA doesn't have a specialty for cosmetic dentistry alone, which means that almost any dentist can say they're a cosmetic dentist by simply taking a few extra courses and in some cases, by simply having a degree from a dental school.

Patients should aim to become educated about the dentist or practice they're going to for cosmetic work, or really for any dental work. Cosmetic dentistry, in reality, requires extensive additional training that isn't offered standard in dental schools. It takes years to learn and perfect techniques and treatments that offer patients the best quality smile.

Every state is different when it comes to requirements for continuing education for dentists. There isn't a firm consistency outside of getting a general degree from a dental college. However, in order to offer patients the very best care and the very best aesthetic outcomes, it really takes years of additional courses, workshops, training, and practice. That's the reason I encourage patients to understand what is required of cosmetic dentists in their state and to really look into what type of background a dentist has before choosing one.

Continuing education is not just a plus - it's really a must when it comes to cosmetic procedures. A dentist doing cosmetic work, in order to get the best results, needs to both understand the technical aspects of the procedures they perform and also be able to visualize the end result before they even begin treatment. I'm incredibly passionate about visualizing a great smile for each of my patients and then giving them the smile I've visualized, the smile they're really looking for.

Cosmetic procedures include not only teeth whitening and veneers, but crowns, teeth shaping, and implants. A number of patients may see an oral surgeon to get the implants and then are passed off to a dentist to get the final dental restorations. The surgeons don't really get to see the end result and how happy the patient is with the aesthetics of their smile. At my practice, we cover both ends, and everything in-between. We visualize the smile, take care of the implants themselves, and then work to shape and shade the teeth attached to the implants to offer our patients the most ideal overall outcome. In more recent years, technology has played a huge role in our ability to perfect these outcomes. We use computers to design the implants and the teeth, to know how and where to place the implants for the most secure and stable bite, and it helps us create natural, beautiful smiles.

WHAT PATIENTS SHOULD BE LOOKING FOR

This might seem slightly repetitive, however, because it is so important, I'd like to address it further. Any patient seeking cosmetic dentistry needs to know, of course, the outcome that they want and make sure that the dentist they choose can offer them that. It's almost impossible to know how good a dentist is without asking questions, doing research on their practice, and talking to other patients who have had work done there. One thing I would always encourage a patient to do is to check for before and after pictures, either online or right in the practice itself. Because of the fact that it does take a lot of time, education, and practice to perfect cosmetic procedures, skilled dentists are happy to show off the before and after photos of the cases they've worked on.

Talk to the dentist. Ask him or her how long they've been doing different procedures, how many of these procedures they've done, and the types of results they've seen. Make sure that the dentist knows exactly what outcome you're looking for and see what type of treatment they recommend to achieve this for you. Ask to talk to other patients. Or if you know people – maybe family or friends – who have been seen at a particular practice, ask them what they had done and how happy they are with their results. It's one thing to get the perspective of the dentist and his associates, but getting feedback from other patients is often an even better way to gauge how happy you'll be if you choose to go with a particular dentist.

COSMETIC DENTISTRY IN THE AGE OF TECHNOLOGY

Technology has become increasingly important in the field of dentistry, and specifically in terms of cosmetic dentistry. In my practice, I'm able to use computers to control almost all of the elements involved. For example, computers are critical in helping to design and place implants. The computer even helps to guide us during the surgery itself. We take 3-D x-rays beforehand to give us a full view of the mouth and jaw.

Aside from surgeries, computers are critical in helping us find and create the ideal shades for teeth, allowing us to custom color match to a patient's existing teeth. This makes their final result more seamless and natural looking. I should mention here that my practice does work hand-in-hand with a lab that is close by. They come to us, help us shape and shade teeth and with other elements used for cosmetic procedures. This has been instrumental in giving my patients their dream smile.

Laser dentistry is another huge part of the technology factor. We use soft tissue lasers in my practice all the time. In the future, we're looking forward to hard tissue lasers. These will inevitably lead to the elimination of tools like drills and other more invasive elements that make a lot of noise and are much messier.

THE FUTURE LAWYER

To wrap up this topic, I'd like to share one more patient story with you.

This case is the one that I remember most, for a number of reasons. The patient I'm talking about was a young man in high school when he came to see me. He had a terrible overbite, sometimes referred to as having "buckteeth". To be completely honest, the worst case I had ever seen. When he bit down, there was almost literally enough space to insert a golf ball.

He'd gone to an orthodontist previous to seeing me and they said they wouldn't take his case. That practice had told him that he'd need surgery where his jaw would be broken and his lower jaw would have to be pulled forward or the upper jaw would have to be pushed back. His parents, at that time, couldn't afford that and it wasn't going to be covered by insurance.

When I saw him, he was really just desperate for some help. He told me that he was constantly made fun of, called every mean name in the book. He was willing to do anything to help correct the problem. I could see that this situation had been causing him huge personal and social insecurity. I knew that I could help him but I let him know that he'd have to trust me and comply with every aspect of the treatment. He was more than willing, one of the most compliant patients I've ever had. I'd told him this because I knew it was going to be an involved, lengthy process, and it was. For three years I worked on his case, promising him only that I'd do the very best I could because I really wanted to help him. In the end, his case turned out beautifully. He was so happy. I was thrilled. I've used his case and models – with his permission – to show to other patients.

What makes this case even more memorable is what happened later. Right after high school, he and his family moved out of the area so I didn't get to see what happened in his life. But then he came back as a patient after fifteen years. He was back in the area practicing as a lawyer. A lawyer!

He told me after all these years he had to come back and find me because after the treatment I and my staff had provided, it boosted his confidence and pushed him to chase his dream of going to law school. He told me how much he loved his beautiful smile, how he'd felt confident to socialize, how he'd made all of these new relationships and pursued and gotten his dream job.

I wanted to share this story because it is a powerful reflection of the dramatic and life-changing effect that a beautiful smile can have on a person's life. His case was not only an issue of structure and cosmetics. It was also a serious case of confidence issues. Ultimately, his case is a prime example of why I do what I do and why I love doing it. I just want all of my patients, at the end of the day, to have the smile of their dreams.

ABOUT DONALD VESPA, DDS

Pinellas Family Dental
www.DentalFlorida.com

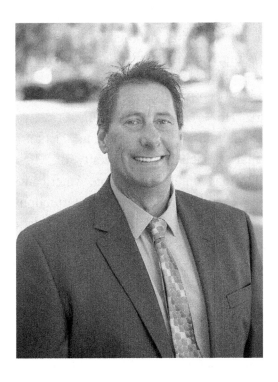

Dr. Don Vespa is a graduate of the University of Missouri at Kansas City School of Dentistry. For more than 30 years, Dr. Vespa practiced in Missouri, operating the Gentle Dental Center in West Branson; today, he and his wife and dental partner, Dr. Amy Vespa, are living their dream in Florida. His love of the outdoors has enabled him and his family to pursue the goal of living in a year-round warm climate, and he now provides top-notch care to patients in the Sunshine State through Pinellas Family Dental.

Dr. Vespa has built a reputation as a dental professional with a comprehensive approach to oral health care, including the use of the latest technology in patient treatment. Dr. Vespa has spent his career developing both diagnostic and therapeutic skills in order to give his patients the best possible care. Dr. Vespa offers treatment in clear orthodontics, endodontics, cosmetic dentistry, laser dentistry and oral surgery. He focuses on developing strong doctor-patient relationships in order to give his patients a truly professional, comprehensive dental experience.

Dr. Vespa has been preferred provider for Invisalign® for the past 14 years. He is also a member of many professional organizations, including the American Dental Association, Missouri Dental Association, University of Missouri Alumni Association, Florida Dental Association, American Straight Wire Orthodontic Association, American Orthodontic Society, Academy of General Dentistry, and Midwest Sedation Dentistry. He was awarded "Best of Tampa Bay" for 2017 by the *Tampa Bay Times* newspaper and was appointed as "Top Cosmetic & Implant Dentist" in Florida for 2017.

Dr. Vespa's attention to the needs of his patients has earned him their trust and respect. With a focus on comfort, convenience and effective treatment, Dr. Vespa offers patients a holistic dental treatment plan that addresses every need, including pain-free dentistry and cosmetic as well as therapeutic results. A resident of Tampa, he and his wife are the proud parents of a new baby, Nikolas, and two Sheltie puppies.

TODAY'S CROWNS ARE INCOGNITO

Having a great smile is important for a number of reasons. I feel it's important to start this chapter by letting readers know that in my practice, our primary purpose and goal is to give patients the very best care, the very best results, and to leave them feeling empowered to tackle their lives. It's also my hope that in doing this, others will take notice and be motivated to seek getting the smile they really want and become empowered as well.

There are many different procedures and techniques used in the field of dentistry to address the problems a person has with their teeth and their smile. Crowns and fillings are two commonly used treatment options to help patients work towards their ideal smile.

EARLY HISTORY OF FILLINGS

The history of fillings can't truly be explored without talking about the reason for their existence. Cavities or holes in the teeth are the root of the creation and existence of fillings. There are specific forms of bacteria that produce acid which destroys tooth enamel and erodes the dentin underneath, causing holes. Some of the earliest papers ever found on dentistry come from 5000 B.C., papers which describe "tooth worms" which caused decay of teeth. While we understand today that there aren't actually "worms", it's safe to assume that this name was chosen because of the holes left behind.

MODERN DENTAL FILLINGS

What we know as modern dentistry and fillings started sometime in the early 16th century, with the most up-to-date research indicating evidence of the practice of using fillings around the year 1530. During this time period, records and artifacts show the use of silver, or more accurately, a silver paste, being used to repair and fill decaying and damaged teeth. Even before this, around 700 A.D., there are articles that reveal the mention and possible use of a similar type of paste in China. However, most research finds the most credible and solid foundation of modern dental fillings starting several hundreds of years later.

AMALGAM FILLINGS

For the last 150 years or so, amalgam fillings have been very popular. Amalgam is a combination of metals. Silver amalgam fillings, one of the most widely used, are actually a combination of silver, mercury, copper, zinc, and palladium. The primary reason for the wide use and popularity of amalgam fillings is likely the abundance of these metals, also because of their durability. The combination of metals could be easily melted down and formed into a mixture that is very malleable, meaning it can be easily manipulated and fit into cavities in a tooth before hardening to its original strength. Gold an alternative, however, because of its expense, most patients and dentists favored the silver amalgam fillings.

Amalgam fillings have fallen out of popularity in recent decades for several reasons. One of the most controversial aspects of these fillings is mercury use. Today more than ever, we understand how detrimental mercury is to a person's health. Aesthetics is another reason. This combination of metals, while durable, isn't the same color as a person's tooth. Depending on where the filling is placed or how many fillings of this type a person has, they can be very visible and thus create dark or discolored spaces in a person's smile. This is a major cosmetic drawback to amalgam fillings.

I don't use amalgam fillings in my practice, however, there are some dentists that do. When I started practicing in 1992, amalgam fillings were rapidly falling out of favor. Even back in my early days of practicing, I remember doing dental work in the military and finding that most of the people I worked on wanted alternative fillings, white restorations that camouflaged the work that had been done. Of course, I want my patients to have the very best smile possible. The alternatives I use in my practice are just as strong and reliable as amalgam fillings, if not more so, and provide my patients with a great looking smile as well.

BETTER COSMETIC ALTERNATIVES TO AMALGAM FILLINGS

Today, with the advances that have been made in the field of dentistry, we do have excellent alternative fillings to offer patients. One of these alternatives is composite resin fillings. These are synthetic resins which take the place of the combination of metals. Porcelain fillings are another option. These can be cast and bonded to the tooth.

These alternatives help to alleviate the problems with amalgam fillings. By eliminating the combination of metals that include mercury, we avoid unnecessary mercury exposure. Also, over time, metal expands, and this can and does create cracks in teeth. I often see patients that have had silver amalgam fillings for a period of time. I noticed because of the amount of force a tooth is subjected to daily, combined with the expansion of the metal fillings, these patients tend to have cracks occurring around their fillings.

Aesthetics is also a huge reason for the use of alternative fillings. In today's society, the constant pursuit of a beautiful, straight, white smile is everywhere. No one wants to intentionally put something dark in their mouth. It sticks out noticeably, now more than ever, in a world where everyone wants 1,000-watt smiles. Using alternative filling and white restoration options make it possible to have the ideal color or shade that a patient is looking for. It camouflages the decay and blends in more seamlessly with a person's natural teeth and their overall smile.

COMPOSITE RESIN VERSUS PORCELAIN FILLINGS

While both composite resin and porcelain fillings are alternatives to amalgam, they each have pros and cons, specifically when compared to one another.

Porcelain can be used for fillings and restorations of a patient's teeth. Porcelain has to be cast. First, an impression of the tooth has to be made. Then, the impression is used by lab technicians to mill and fabricate the porcelain that will then be bonded to the patient's tooth. Because of its beautiful aesthetic quality, as well as the amount of work that goes into making and bonding the porcelain, it is generally more expensive than composite resin filling treatment.

Composite restorations are more affordable than porcelain, however, they tend to leak over time once they are used. In some cases, they can stain a patient's teeth and in certain cases, they have to be replaced. Even with patients who have excellent oral hygiene, who clean their teeth and have regular checkups, composite restorations will often fail and the patient will have to have them replaced.

Porcelain restorations generally have a stronger bond than composite resin restorations, making them more durable and long-lasting. Also, as previously mentioned, their aesthetic quality is better. Because they are created by lab technicians, people who are true artists when it comes to fabricating and creating the restorations, they mimic the hills and grooves of a real tooth, keeping the restoration true to the patient's natural teeth. The color and shading of the restoration will fit in with the patient's natural teeth so that the restoration is basically invisible.

CROWNS

Crowns are different than fillings because they cover the tooth, mimicking the original shape and color of the existing, damaged tooth. In cases where the patient's tooth has been severely compromised and is in need of significant restoration, crowns are the best option.

Crowns are also made from different materials than fillings. They offer a variety of crowns, including gold, zirconium, ceramics, and some crowns are made with base metal alloys. Today, we mostly use zirconium crowns and ceramic crowns because they are white and are therefore more aesthetically pleasing.

Ceramic crowns are generally used for front teeth because they are most visible. Ceramic crowns are made of porcelain base materials, which is why they are white. Zirconium crowns are also favorable because zirconium is what we would consider a white metal. These crowns are very popular because of their ability to bind to teeth and to withstand the forces of grinding, chewing, and any other action that requires a person to put pressure on their teeth. In fact, zirconium is really a great base metal to use to bind ceramic crowns because it easily bonds and stabilizes the porcelain in the ceramic crown. There are a variety of porcelain and ceramic crowns used today. These are generally the most aesthetically pleasing because they are translucent, allowing light to pass through them and make them look very natural.

THE LIFE OF A CROWN

When I attended dental school, it was recommended – with what we knew about basic and dental materials involved in making crowns – to tell patients that crowns typically last about 10 years. There are a lot of variables with each patient that can change the length of the life of a crown. Great oral hygiene and regular checkups can lead to crowns lasting significantly longer, or you might need to have crowns replaced in 2 years, or 5 years. It truly just depends on the individual patient.

Patients who take excellent care of their teeth might be able to keep their crowns for 20 years, or even longer. In fact, I once had a patient who had an entire bridge of crowns that had come loose, 12 units – or crowns/teeth – that we were preparing to replace. I told her that I'd need to tap the bridge to see if it was stable structurally and also check the status of the teeth underneath. It's important to note that replacing the entire bridge would have cost this patient tens of thousands of dollars.

When I took her bridge out and checked it, it was in excellent shape. We cleaned it and examined the teeth she had under the bridge. They were in good shape as well. Because of this, I was able to simply re-cement her existing bridge. She literally said,

"Whooh! Dr. Pagan, you are a god." I told her, of course, that I was not a god, and that her taking good care of her teeth was the main reason I was able to keep the necessary repair work to a minimum. She'd taken excellent care of her teeth and her bridge for 30 years. The bridge bonding had simply come loose after wear and tear over those years and was easily put back into place. I remember this case specifically because it was so unusual and because it left me feeling so good about being able to easily fix the problem.

How Crowns Are Made

Dental crowns are most often carefully crafted by hand. This can't usually be done in the dentist's office. Instead, it is done in a dental laboratory. Before crowns can be placed, the patient's teeth have to be prepared, removing decay and creating a solid shape with what is left of the natural tooth. Then an impression is made so the crown can be formed around the shape of the tooth that it will be bonded to. Because the teeth don't look their best once they've been prepared for a crown, we make a temporary crown that the patient can wear for a few weeks until the permanent crown is made. Once the patient comes back for the follow-up visit, the temporary crown is removed and the permanent crown is bonded to the patient's tooth. During the time that the patient is wearing the temporary crown, the lab is using the impressions and any x-rays that were taken to create the true crown that will be bonded to the patient's tooth.

Crowns: Labs versus Technology

Technology has come a long way over the past few decades. Enter the CEREC system. This entire technological system can be used to create a variety of things, including crowns. This system uses a computer to scan the tooth. The computer and its software then copy this and then the CEREC machine actually makes the crown. One of the great advantages of this system is that it produces the crown promptly so that it can be bonded to the patient's tooth in one visit.

I don't have this technology in my office, but I know a lot of dentists who do. Today, the crowns that are made using the CEREC system can look just as good as those created in a dental lab. However, I am still personally partial to the hands-on approach, creating and sculpting the crown manually, which allows us more freedom to play around with colors and shading.

A TOTAL TRANSFORMATION

I'd like to share a story, a case that I worked on which shows how transformative crowns can be.

A woman in her 60s came to see me. She'd suffered from spousal abuse and had gone through very difficult times. She had let her teeth go and they'd begun to decay significantly. She was terribly embarrassed by how her teeth looked. She hated the discoloration that the decay had caused. She also had some composite restorations that had begun to leak and cause stains as well. She avoided smiling and when she talked, she often tried to cover her mouth.

I mentioned to her that I could use several crowns – otherwise known as an arch – to totally fix her smile. I let her know that we had to use arches because she needed multiple crowns and doing one at a time would make it impossible to match the structure of her mouth and teeth, and it would make it extremely difficult to match colors accurately so that one or two crowns didn't stand out from the rest. I ended up doing a full restoration of her entire mouth. We'd prepared her teeth and given her the temporary crowns she needed to wear, partially for aesthetic reasons, and because they provide a more solid base so that she would be able to chew and her teeth would fit together correctly.

She came back to get her true crowns put in. When we were done and she looked in the mirror, she began to cry. These were genuine tears of happiness and, I think, shock at how great her smile looked. "Wow," she said. "This is the smile I had when I was younger. This is exactly how my smile looked then." It was wonderful and amazing to hear her response and to see how completely transformed her smile was. I worked with the lab technicians who sculpted and created these crowns. They are works of art that transform the way a person looks. This is why I love doing what I do.

INLAYS AND ONLAYS VERSUS FILLINGS AND CROWNS

Fillings and crowns aren't the only options to correct tooth decay. Inlays and onlays can be compared to fillings and crowns, however, they are used for different cases.

Inlays are typically reserved for cavities that are more severe than those where fillings are used but not so severe that a crown is needed. The decay, of course, must first be removed. The next step also reveals another significant difference between inlays and fillings: the type of material that is used. Fillings, as I mentioned earlier, are typically amalgam or composite resin. An inlay, on the other hand, is a single, solid piece generally created by a lab, though in some practices they can be created in the dentist's office. These pieces are usually created using gold or ceramic.

Inlays also usually take longer, involving multiple visits, because the inlay must be designed to fit the exact space that has been created by removing the cavity or decay from the tooth. If the piece doesn't fit perfectly, food and bacteria can creep into the tooth and create further damage and decay. The major upside to inlays is that they don't contract as much as fillings do, meaning there is a far greater likelihood that this type of restoration won't fail and need to be fixed or replaced. The downside to inlays is that they are more expensive and they aren't frequently used because of the cost and the fact that most insurance won't cover them.

Onlays are more involved and are closer to dental crowns. In fact, they're sometimes referred to as a "partial crown". Onlays are typically reserved for patients who have larger areas of decay, a situation where a filling or an inlay isn't an option. Onlays, unlike inlays, cover the entire cusp of the tooth, the biting surface, while inlays fill the area between cusps. Onlays must be carefully designed and fitted to match the exact space where decay has been removed. Crowns, on the other hand, cover the entire biting surface as well as the rest of the tooth structure that sits above the gum line.

Onlays are less aggressive than crowns. Costs tend to be fairly similar but onlays are usually the less expensive option. Many dentists try to use onlays first, before resorting to crowns, because they are less involved and require less invasion of the natural tooth. The downside is that onlays are much more difficult to do correctly and their success depends entirely on the experience and skill of the dentist. The other caveat is that, like inlays, onlays aren't frequently covered by insurance. Because crowns are covered by most insurance, they have gained a lot of favor with dentists and patients and are therefore more frequently used.

A Very Personal Smile Transformation

I'd like to share one final story with you. This particular case is very personal for me because the patient I worked on is my mother.

My mother had some significant decay and other issues with her smile. Before she came in to see me, she'd been taking care of her husband, and he had recently passed away. Once she'd dealt with that, she came in to get what would be a complete smile transformation. The truth is that I'm still working on her, doing implants and limits ortho on her lower crown arch. However, a short time ago, I was able to give her an upper arch and several veneers and crowns. In all honesty, the transformation was amazing. She was thrilled and loved the way it looked. To me, it was like winning the lottery, being able to give her a truly beautiful smile. I'd wanted to do this for her for quite awhile, but, because she was taking care of her husband, it just wasn't feasible.

Of course, I want to give every single one of my patients this same experience and I'm thrilled each and every time a patient is overjoyed with how their smile looks. But in this particular case, seeing my mom moved to joyful tears is one of the biggest victories I've experienced as a dentist.

The Beauty of Transformative Dentistry

I do a lot of things in my practice to give my patients the smile they're looking for. At the end of the day, what I really do, or what I and my office strive to do, is change the lives of my patients. Whether it's one or two teeth at a time, or multiple teeth, what we actually do here is remove the patient's physical pain, emotional distress, and embarrassment, and boost their confidence and motivation by giving them a winning smile.

Also, as I mentioned at the beginning of the chapter, this transformation affects not only them but everyone they interact with. It's always my hope that someone who's suffering from unresolved dental issues will interact with one of my patients, then come and see me or another dentist and start down the path to get the smile they've been dreaming of. Doing this work doesn't just help my patients. I always thank them for letting me be of assistance because by helping them, I believe I become a better person. Every case, every success story, every transformation changes my life for the better, too. This is the heart of why I do what I do.

ABOUT ERICK V. PAGAN, DMD

Pagan Affinity Dentistry
www.PaganAffinityDentistry.com

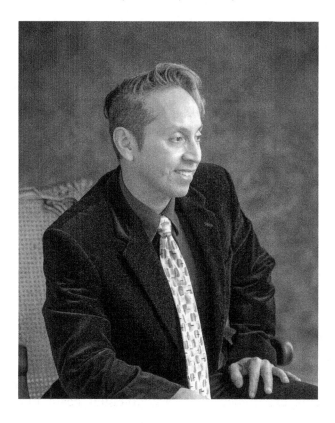

Dr. Erick V. Pagan became interested in dentistry at a very young age, after noticing how his grandmother's face improved when she put in her dentures. By the time he was 8 years old, he knew he wanted to become a dentist.

Dr. Pagan pursued his dream by studying hard. He even skipped a grade in order to enter college earlier. After pursuing an undergraduate degree in pre-dental and graduating *cum laude*, he attended dental school at The Medical College of Georgia. He attended graduate school in 1991 and practiced for two years at

Fort Gordon military base. In 1995, Dr. Pagan purchased a private practice in Washington, Georgia. He purchased another practice and combined the two to form a dental specialty practice in 2006.

Today, Dr. Pagan provides much-needed specialist care for those in the Washington, Georgia, area. Before he bought these practices, many patients in the area had to drive more than an hour to see a specialist. Because he realizes the responsibility he has to the people of his community, Dr. Pagan challenges himself to learn and expand his skills in all areas of dental practice.

Today, Dr. Pagan and his team offer comprehensive dental care including full mouth reconstruction, Invisalign® and Clear Correct Braces, bridges, inlay and onlays, porcelain and full noble crowns, implant placement and crown abutments, laser dentistry, oral cancer screening, periodontal therapy, root canal therapy, tooth extractions with bone replacement therapy, smile makeovers, veneers, whitening, cleaning and always looking for the newest and most updated technology to bring to his patients and treating a wide range of other treatments. Dr. Pagan treats his patients as he does his own family. His loving and compassionate dental care enables him to be ready to take on any dental situation and help his patients experience their best potential heath through his comprehensive treatment plans.

FIFTY SHADES OF WHITE

Having a great smile communicates a lot of things, especially in the society that we live in today. It says a great deal to others – based purely on appearance – about how a person values themselves, and about how capable they are, namely, in terms of taking care of themselves. Often, having a brilliant white smile is a huge part of the overall concern over appearance. Completing cosmetic procedures for patients – such as teeth whitening – is one way that I can help my patients change how they are perceived, both by others and by themselves. At the end of the day, having a beautiful smile is about so much more than just aesthetics. It's a tool that drastically impacts how my patients feel and how successfully they function in all the various facets of their lives.

LET ME START WITH A STORY

I'd like to start with a brief story about one patient who saw a distinct turnaround in his life after getting his teeth whitened.

The patient I'm talking about was in his late forties or right around 50 at the time that I saw him. He had a fairly high-profile job working in the community as an individual involved with the government. He came to me and told me how people often would make fun of him and joke about the fact that his smile was kind of dull and just not that great. After he received his whitening treatment, he came back to my office and told me, "No one has said anything negative about my smile since the treatment. In fact, I've actually received nothing but compliments on it now." As a government employee, working in cities and in front of powerful and influential people, as well as in front of cameras, he was constantly being seen and was clearly bothered by the way his smile was criticized. The whitening treatment shut the jokes down and let him get on with business, with a big smile on his face.

THE CAUSES OF TEETH DISCOLORATION

One of the most common and fairly obvious causes of tooth discoloration is surface stains. These stains are picked up over the natural course of a patient's life and predominantly occur in individuals who consume significantly large amounts of things like coffee, tea, soda, and red wine. Any products that are heavily pigmented are therefore harsh on peoples' teeth. Most people aren't aware of how porous teeth are, which means that they are really good at soaking up colors from whatever the person consumes.

Over time, the bumps, grooves, valleys, and little "potholes" on the surface of a person's teeth pick up stains that then cause a yellowing, darkening, or other discoloration of a person's smile. Patients with surface stains are much easier to treat and generally have more successful experiences with whitening services. In my experience, I'm able to give these types of patients a significantly whiter smile, five or more shades whiter in some cases. In recent years, it seems that the consumption of coffees, different juices, and other pigment-laden ingredients has risen, which is largely the reason why I feel like I have a lot more patients coming in for whitening treatments to alleviate surface stains.

There are a wide variety of things that can and do lead to teeth discoloration. It can start well before a person is born, resulting from how a mother cares for her own body while carrying a child. Mothers who took tetracycline while pregnant often end up having discoloration of their own teeth and, when their children are born, the kids also have discolored teeth. This is because tetracycline gets into the child's tooth structure as it is being formed. Tetracycline is an antibiotic used to treat a variety of infections. In the late 1970s and early 1980s, tetracycline was commercially popular and used extensively to treat individuals with acne. However, one of the predominant side effects of this drug, especially when children are exposed before birth, is internal banding and dark discoloration of the teeth. Unfortunately, patients with discoloration as a result of tetracycline are some of the most difficult cases to treat. The use of tetracycline, because of this and other side effects, has dropped significantly in recent years and is widely avoided for patients that are pregnant.

It's also important to note that age plays a pretty significant role in the discoloration of a person's teeth. Younger patients often see a much more drastic and lasting effect from whitening treatments. Older patients' teeth can be a little more resistant to whitening treatments because of the years of wear and tear and staining.

My practice is adult-based, which means the patients that I treat are 18 or older. When it comes to the average age of patients looking for whitening treatments, it varies widely, although I'd say that the majority of the patients that I personally see are in their thirties and forties.

When Whitening Treatments are Desired

In most cases, a patient seeks a whitening treatment because they are seeking a change or are preparing to enter into a change in their lives and want the added boost they feel from having a beautiful white smile. In many cases, I see older patients who are coming in to whiten their smile because their children or grandchildren have said something to them about their teeth or because they are preparing for an event like a graduation or wedding and the patient wants to have a nice smile for photos. The same is true for people who are switching careers mid-life, going back to school, or heading into a career after graduating. I also see a lot of individuals who are coming out of a divorce or the breakup of a long-term relationship and want a nice, white smile as they get back out into the dating world. The common theme is a major life change.

Whitening is also very common after the removal of braces. Many times, I get questions – especially from parents – about whether or not it's too early to start whitening treatments. Most kids having braces or getting braces off are around 15 or 16, and, there is really no harm in doing it then. In my practice, once a patient has finished with their braces, we do a complimentary whitening treatment to freshen up their smile and help them celebrate the milestone. Traditional braces – because of the metal bands and brackets that get in the way of proper cleaning – tend to lead to more stains and leftover residue, which, of course, I always clean off first before doing any whitening treatments. Invisalign® trays, because they are removable, make it easier for patients to maintain their oral hygiene. Still, I believe it's a great way to help the patient feel more confident, after going through the somewhat lengthy task of straightening their teeth, to offer them an even brighter smile.

TYPES OF WHITENING TREATMENTS

There are a lot of over-the-counter treatments available that patients should know about. I'm not crazy about a lot of the whitening toothpastes because what I've seen, in my experience, is patients using toothpastes that actually have some abrasive elements which scrape away a little bit of the outer layer of the teeth. While this can provide some whitening effect, it's not the most ideal way to achieve that goal. There are also, of course, whitening strips that can be applied at home for a small amount of improvement.

The next type of treatment would be what I would call a small exposure whitening after a full dental cleaning. This type of treatment is performed in the office. For many years, Zoom Whitening was the go-to thing for this type of whitening treatment. After facing some sensitivity concerns with patients, we've switched to the Sinsational Whitening system. This is essentially a preloaded tray, filled with gel, that is placed in the patient's mouth and activated with a special light. This treatment only takes about thirty minutes and is really used as a booster after the patient's teeth have been professionally cleaned. It's fairly mild and can offer a two to three-shade difference in tooth color.

The third type of whitening treatment is more intensive and is really designed for the patient who's looking for a more aggressive and transformative whitening experience. For this treatment, the patient comes in for a visit and has impressions of their mouth made so that we can build trays designed to precisely fit the specific aspects of the person's mouth. This allows for a more secure fit and a better overall whitening in the end. Once the trays are ready, we provide patients with the trays and the whitening gel to take home, enough for about two weeks of treatments. This system is designed to create one hour of exposure to the whitening gel per day, generally thirty minutes in the morning and thirty minutes at night.

The final whitening treatment to mention, and the one I personally believe is most effective, is something called Kor Whitening. This system is a totally different approach and requires a lot of commitment on the part of the patient. The Kor trays are designed not only to fit the patient, but also to seal off the gel from coming too far up and connecting with the gums, which is often what leads to a lot of patient sensitivity. This also prevents oxygen from getting to the gel while it's whitening, which means it can remain effective for six hours or more. There is an in-office treatment, and then the patient wears the trays overnight for a minimum of two weeks. Once the gel portion of the treatment is done, the patient comes back to the office and has a half hour power bleaching session to finish off the treatment. The results from the Kor treatments are truly incredible and often don't require a significant amount of follow up because the teeth tend to stay white.

THE KOR SYSTEM IN ACTION

Before I continue talking about the ins-and-outs of whitening treatments, I'd like to share the story of one of my patients.

I saw a girl, one of my younger patients, in her early twenties. She was just out of college and was on the hunt for her career. She had a yellowish smile but didn't really have the time, money, or desire for porcelain teeth or veneers. In reality, she had nice, straight teeth, they just needed to be "refreshed". She decided to go with the Kor whitening treatment and, by the end, I have to say that she was very impressed and even I was blown away by the amazing difference it made to her smile and how beautiful and white her teeth were. She was able to head out into the working work with a bright, white, gorgeous smile.

WHITENING TREATMENTS ARE SAFE

As whitening treatments have become more and more common, we've seen through studies and research not only how effective they are, but how safe they can be. The key factor in the safety, however, is doing it properly and with advice from a professional. As I mentioned before, patients can experience a great deal of sensitivity when the whitening gel they use gets all over their gums. There is also, of course, sometimes sensitivity to the teeth. However, this can be easily stopped and even prevented with special toothpaste designed for sensitive teeth. The sensitive teeth are also often a result of improper usage of and exposure to the whitening gel. Different treatments are designed to be worn for specific periods of time. It's generally the patients who don't follow directions properly, or who end up with their teeth exposed for too long to the gel, that end up with sensitivity issues. The key to making sure that your whitening experience goes smoothly is to make sure to talk to a professional and follow the directions you're given with any follow-up or at-home care.

HOW LONG WHITENING TREATMENTS LAST

The length of time that a whitening treatment lasts depends a lot on what type of treatment a patient has done and how they care for their teeth, which includes diet. If you consume a lot of red wine, coffee, tea, or any types of foods or beverages that are known to stain teeth, you'll need to get a booster whitening treatment more often. I generally recommend that patients who get trays for whitening treatments keep their trays and get another tube of gel when they come in for a cleaning so that they can do a booster treatment the same day. For the average person, I generally recommend a booster treatment every six months or around the time they'd usually come in for a cleaning. However, if their diet is heavy in foods and drinks that stain their teeth, then they might need to do a booster treatment more often.

This is slightly different with the Kor whitening system. With the Kor system, I've seen very little rebounding in stains with my patients. There is always, of course, a little bit of staining that occurs over time, however, most patients that undergo a Kor treatment see a drastic shade change – up to 10 shades lighter – with very little relapse even after a long period of time without a booster treatment.

It's important to remember that the actual shade difference a patient sees is dependent upon the type of treatment they have and maintaining it depends on how they care for their teeth afterward. It's also important to note that you will, at some point, reach the whitest shade you're going to get. And while booster whitening treatments are a great way to maintain your white smile, continuing to do it for years and years on end isn't always necessary and can become excessive.

WHEN ARE WHITENING TREATMENTS NOT IN THE CARDS?

There are definitely circumstances that would take a patient out of the running for whitening treatments. Pregnant women should not get whitening treatments. Anything you put into your mouth and your body could be passed along to the growing baby. The same goes for mothers who are nursing. These chemicals can enter the mother's system and be transferred through breastmilk.

Whitening treatments are also not recommended for patients who can't or won't follow directions. This goes back to what I was talking about earlier in this chapter. All of the whitening treatment methods come with some form of instruction and some level of commitment on the patient's part. If the patient can't follow these directions – or doesn't want to – they could ultimately cause themselves harm in the process.

Whitening treatments should also not be used on really young patients and small children. These children's bodies, gums, teeth, and jaws are all still growing and developing. Also, the majority of the teeth that would be whitening are most likely the child's primary teeth which are going to fall out to make way for their permanent teeth, meaning the whitening process would be entirely lost in a short amount of time.

One final thing to note in this section is the matter of people with veneers, crowns, fillings, bondings, or anything in their mouth that isn't just their natural teeth. If they attempt to whiten their teeth at home without the assistance of a professional, they will end up with less than satisfactory results because only the natural teeth will be whitened. If you have any of these elements in your mouth, you're not excluded from whitening treatments, however, it's best to seek help from a professional for the best results. It's generally best to get whitening treatments done first and then get crowns, fillings, and the like put in place afterward so that they can be matched to the current shade of your teeth.

WHAT IT COSTS TO WHITEN YOUR TEETH

It's important to know, from the beginning, that teeth whitening treatments are purely cosmetic and therefore there isn't something that an insurance company or plan that will cover, so all of the cost will come straight out of your pocket. This is something to keep in mind when considering the variety of options there are available to you.

The actual cost of different treatments – those offered by dentists and not over-the-counter – varies by the area of the country you're in and the skill and experience level of the doctor providing you the treatments. Let me first talk, specifically, about the treatments offered at my practice. With the Sinsational Whitening system, you're looking around $99. If you want to get the custom whitening trays – which you can keep and reuse for boosters down the road – you'll pay about $250 for that whitening treatment. The Kor whitening system is the most expensive because of the amount of time you have to spend in the office, the cost of the materials, and the fabrication of the highly-specialized trays. In my practice, we're right around the $1,400 mark for a full Kor system treatment.

The reality is that you really get what you pay for. Yes, over-the-counter whitening strips are usually under $100. However, you're likely only going to see a shade or two difference in terms of whitening power. Then, of course, as you step up in the intensity of commitment and shade difference potential with each treatment, you also step up in price. The important thing is to discuss what results you're looking for with your dentist, talk about what you can financially handle, and work together to figure out which treatment is most feasible and cost-effective for you.

ONE LAST STORY

There's one final patient story I'd like to share with you.

I had a patient, a nice gentleman who decided, after consulting with me, to use the Kor whitening system. As I established earlier in the chapter, tetracycline usage is something that can cause discoloration of the teeth. This man had used tetracycline earlier in his life and he had a fair number of dark bands and general discoloration of his teeth after years of wear, tear, and stains. After we used the Kor treatment, he saw a drastic and really nice color change. The great thing about this man's case is that we were able to drastically improve the brightness and evenness of his smile – in terms of color – with the whitening treatment instead of having to resort to the much more invasive and costly treatment of porcelain veneers. He was very happy with the results, and we were very happy with the results.

All of the stories I've shared in this chapter paint a great picture of exactly what whitening treatments can do for a person. Whether you're preparing for a new venture in life, starting a new career, getting married, graduating from school, or even if you're just getting your braces off, a great whitening treatment can enhance your teeth and improve your confidence in your smile. At the end of the day, it's really about changing people's lives by boosting their confidence and helping them feel better about themselves and what they can accomplish. That's the beauty of helping someone get the nice, white smile that they're looking for.

About Wayne Sutton, DDS

Sonoma Smiles

www.SonomaSmiles.com

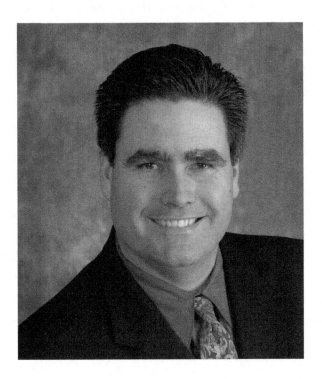

Dr. Wayne Sutton has been recognized as one of Sonoma County's premier cosmetic dentists. A graduate of The Pacific Aesthetic Continuum in San Francisco, he also studied Advanced Occlusion at the prestigious Hornbrook Group.

Dr. Sutton received his DDS in 1997 from UCSF School of Dentistry, where he also spent three years as a clinical instructor. He was the only recipient of the coveted "Clinical Excellence Award" in 1997. In 2006, Dr. Sutton became one of the first dentists in Northern California to earn his Fellowship in the Academy of Comprehensive Esthetics. Each year, he completes more than four times the required professional development courses in California in order to broaden his knowledge of advances in dental procedures.

Dr. Sutton is an active member of American Academy of Cosmetic Dentistry and the American Dental Association. He holds fellowships in the Dental Organization for Conscious Sedation, the Academy of General Dentistry, and the American Dental Implant Association. Dr. Sutton is also a member of the American Academy for Dental Sleep Medicine.

One of Dr. Sutton's goals is to educate the public about the dangers of sleep apnea and offer testing and treatment options. He often gives lectures to local groups about dental technology and cosmetic dentistry.

Dr. Sutton has appeared on KFTY News Channel 50 as the local expert in cosmetic dentistry. He is also a regional consultant for dental related questions through his website at www.sonomasmiles.com. His office offers digital photography for the best patient outcomes, and he also helps teach other dental professionals how to incorporate digital photography into their practices.

Dr. Sutton has produced and manufactured an educational DVD entitled "Simplified Smile Design." He is one of a select group of cosmetic dentists to be recognized as an Official Dentist of the Mrs. Globe – Mrs. USA Pageants. Most recently, Dr. Sutton has become the franchise owner of Teeth Tomorrow Sonoma County, through which he helps people who need full mouth dental implant reconstructions using the strongest dental implant bridge available today. Information can be found at www.teethtomorrowsonomacounty.com.

THE FOUNDATION OF A GREAT SMILE

There are a variety of gum issues that a person can have, many of which affect the way a person looks. With a multitude of teeth and bone issues, people often forget – or don't even realize – how much a gum problem can affect how their smile looks, or the significant effects it can have on the overall health of their mouth.

GUM PRESENTATION AND HEALTH

One of the first issues I'd like to address when it comes to gums is presentation. Everyone has a gingival biotype – how their gums naturally present or look. I often refer to these biotypes as gum 'personalities'. Some individuals have a thin gum personality. Patients with this type of gum personality generally have thinner gum tissue, which can be more likely to recede away from the teeth. These patients also generally have ovoid, longer, and more slender shaped teeth. In most cases, we tend to see this more commonly in female patients than in male patients.

The second biotype, or personality, is what we commonly refer to as thick gums. The gum tissue here is thicker where it meets the tooth and typically results in the teeth appearing more square in shape. Thicker tissues are firm and bound to the underlying bone which presents a flatter arch appearance. As a contrast to the previous gum personality, thick gums are viewed as more masculine because men tend to have this presentation more than women.

Sometimes, however, thick gum tissue is an issue of swelling, which can be caused by gingivitis. Poor oral hygiene is often the culprit when it comes to this, but it's not the only concern. Thick gums can also be caused by certain medications or a combination of medications. We can also find thicker, fibrotic gum tissue in patients who smoke. Before this can be treated, we have to get to the root of the cause. Depending on what the specific issue is for each patient, we can recommend medication changes – of course with the input of the doctor or doctors who prescribed them – provide assistance with smoking cessation, and also give patients an updated education on how to care for their teeth properly.

The health of a patient's gum tissue is really important for the patient's overall health but it also plays a large role in how appealing the person's smile is. Healthy gum tissue is nice and pink, and doesn't show signs of swelling. Red, swollen, or otherwise visibly infected tissue indicates underlying problems with the gums that need to be addressed. If the patient has otherwise naturally appealing gums, treating any gum tissue disease will allow their natural gum presentation and beauty to shine through.

SOME GUM DISEASE BASICS

There isn't one single dental term to refer to gum disease because there are different types of diseases and different stages. Primarily, we're talking about gingivitis, which, in the simplest of terms, is a disease of the gums that causes them to bleed.

Periodontitis is a different, more severe entity that can be a manifestation of untreated gingivitis. Periodontitis, if left untreated, ends up causing bone and tooth loss in patients.

The reality in America is that a lot of patients have gum disease and are totally unaware of it. Recent studies with the National Health and Nutrition Examination Survey (NHANES) – conducted by the National Center for Health Statistics (NCHS) – indicated that more than 80% of the country's population age 30 and older have at least one place in their mouth being impacted by periodontitis. These numbers are referring to chronic periodontitis. There's actually research that reveals a smaller subset of patients who have what we refer to as aggressive periodontitis and unfortunately, a lot of these patients are younger than 30. With these patients, we recognize that immediate and comprehensive treatment is necessary in order to preserve their teeth. This smaller subset of patients, which sits right around 10% of the population, must have the aggressive gum disease treated immediately or they run the risk of more extensive bone and tooth loss.

A 'GUMMY' SMILE

When considering thicker gum tissue medication and hygiene issues are the easiest to treat. Working with patients' physicians to change medications or proper home care instructions will reduce swelling and improve the overall appearance. What is more challenging is working with genetic components that can affect gum tissue thickness and/or how much gum a person shows when they smile. This is generally referred to as a "Gummy Smile" and can happen as a result of a skeletal concern, where the person's upper jaw fits in relation to their face and skull, altered passive eruption, when the teeth don't fully penetrate the arch of their jaw and are partially covered by gum and bone, or in patients who are genetically predisposed to having a shorter upper lip or a hypermobile lip. All three of these concerns result in a wide smile that shows lots of gum.

TREATING A GUMMY SMILE

Treating a patient who presents with a particularly gummy smile first involves determining what the specific cause – or combination of causes – is. The treatments can range from less invasive to more invasive, depending on what specific issues a patient has. If we're dealing with altered passive eruption – where teeth don't fully come into the arch – then we can do a procedure called crown lengthening. This treatment involves reducing some of the gum and even sometimes the bone to show more tooth. There's also a newer procedure called lip repositioning that can be an option for patients with skeletal issues. While the crown lengthening works for the teeth themselves, lip repositioning is really a matter of adjusting where the lip sits, allowing it to hide some of the gum tissue that you'd otherwise see when the patient smiles.

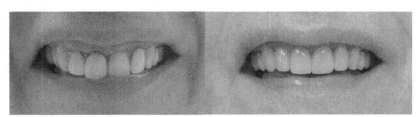

Before and after crown lengthening

In the majority of the cases we treat, we see the best results from either of these first two treatment options or even a combination of the two. For more extensive skeletal and anatomical issues, orthognathic surgery might be required to reposition a patient's jaw, setting it into proper alignment with the person's face and thereby adjusting the amount of gum that is revealed when the person smiles.

THIN GUM BIOTYPES

Individuals with thinner gums and more "toothy" smiles are generally individuals that have had some type of gum recession, and potentially even bone loss, depending on the severity of the case. With the recession of the soft gum tissue, we find that a person's teeth begin to look longer, which can result in an older appearance. This upsets the balance of pink tissue versus white tissue when we look at the smile. For patients with a significant amount of recession, it can look as though their smile is all teeth. Along with this we see an exposing of the space between the teeth, which often looks like dark spots or triangles in the person's mouth and can be confused with food or decay.

Leaving this condition untreated can cause a number of issues for patients besides just an overall displeasure with the way their smile looks. One of the first things we usually find with patients like this is an increased sensitivity to temperature. They often struggle with, or have significant discomfort with, eating or drinking extremely cold or hot foods and beverages. This is can be the first symptom patients voice to their providers.

As gum tissue recedes and exposes the root of a person's tooth, there is a concern with root decay. Cementum, which is the material that teeth roots are made of, isn't as strong as the enamel on a tooth. This means that patients who don't typically have problems with cavities can find themselves at risk for decay as the root tissue is exposed. When gum recession gets to the most drastic and severe points, we find patients suffer tooth looseness. This can result in the loss of teeth from inadequate gum and bone tissue providing support.

TREATING PATIENTS WITH RECEDING GUMS

If recession of the gums is caught early enough, there are a variety of soft tissue grafting techniques we can use to cover up the roots of teeth that have been exposed. Traditional soft tissue grafting involves taking a portion of the tissue from the roof of a patient's mouth and transplanting it around the teeth that are exposed.

There have also been a lot of scientific advances in recent years that enable us to use donor tissue for grafting. This procedure, while it may seem a bit scary, is completely safe and reliable. We get tissue from certified tissue banks that screen donors for any types of diseases, making certain that the tissue is safe to use with the patient it's being implanted in. This also makes it easier on the patient, as they don't have to have two sites impacted by the procedure; they simply have tissue implanted around the affected teeth without having the secondary wound on the roof of their mouth.

Another procedure that prevents taking tissue from the roof of the mouth is a newer procedure known as the pinhole technique. We are able to cover the roots of a patient's teeth without using tissue from the roof of the mouth or having to use donor tissue. The options that involve less trauma to the patient's mouth are, of course, the first options we consider because they are easier on the patient and allow them to heal quicker.

We also can graft hard tissue for patients who not only have gum recession but bone loss as well. In these cases, we are fortunate to have donor tissue that can be used to regrow the lost bone tissue, and then if necessary, we repair the gum recession.

The course of treatment we choose – and how long the treatment process takes – is unique to each patient. Depending on the severity of tissue loss, donor tissue is a really great option when there is minimal loss of tissue volume that affects multiple teeth. If the patient has a great deal of tissue loss – hard or soft – it's usually best to use their own tissue to prevent having to repeat this process down the road.

One of the questions that is frequently asked at consultation visits is how long will treatment take? It's hard to put an estimate on how long it takes to treat each case because every case is different. In the average patient where, for example, only a few teeth need to be treated, the procedure itself can take about 45 minutes to an hour. In terms of post-operative treatment and healing, we find that swelling and discomfort generally peak a few days after the procedure. The further past this peak the patient gets, the better they feel. In most cases, after four or five days, patients start getting back to their normal diet and daily routines.

We encourage all patients – regardless of what procedure they've had done – to take it easy for the first 48 hours. Heavy lifting, strenuous exercise, or anything that involves pressure in the mouth, such as drinking through a straw or smoking, can lead to increased swelling and pain. Some patients can return to work the day after their procedure, but it depends entirely on the type of work that they do and also on them slowing down their pace while working. For patients who have more extensive recession and need more extensive treatment, the length of the procedure and the length of the recovery time pretty much doubles. The goal is to make sure that patients don't put unnecessary stress on themselves. We also recommend anti-inflammatory medication. Ice is also recommended for the first few days to combat swelling and help with pain.

A Special Patient

I'd like to share the story of one of my favorite patients here. His story is a good example of how gum disease can negatively impact your smile and your life.

J is a truck driver I've been seeing for almost ten years now. When he first came to us, he was an uncontrolled diabetic and heavy smoker. He came in because he had difficulty maintaining regular care of his teeth due to his job, and he'd noticed that his four front teeth were starting to develop spaces between them. Because he hadn't been in for regular care for almost five years, he went to his general dentist first with his concern. After seeing the severity of his condition, his dentist told him that he needed to see a periodontist, a doctor that specializes in treating gum disease and related issues.

When J finally came to us, we did a complete exam and found that he did, in fact, have extensive periodontal concerns. His four front teeth were developing spaces between them because of bone loss. There were also concerns with gum recession in his lower arch. We did some general periodontal treatment and performed a procedure called root planning, which is a more in-depth cleaning that enables us to get rid of the staining and tartar build up on teeth and root surfaces. This also helped with the overall color of his gums. We did end up removing the four front teeth that were spaced apart and loose. We placed implants so that he could have a four-unit bridge on two implants, replacing the teeth that were lost. We also used some tissue grafting for his upper teeth so that we could shorten the appearance of the teeth that had been overexposed by the recession of his gums.

The final results were really beautiful. With the combination of treatment techniques, we were able to balance out his smile.

Perhaps the most rewarding aspect about J's case is that once we addressed his oral health and smile issues, he really began to get other aspects of his life in order. He was able to get his diabetes in check, which made his endocrinologist extremely happy, and he also cut back significantly in terms of his smoking. It was really a total transformation. His improved smile and appearance boosted his confidence. When I first started treating him, he didn't make eye contact much, he kept his hat on and pulled down over his face, and he didn't smile. After his treatment was complete, he had an entirely new take on his life and confidence in himself. He found pride in improving the other parts of his health and life that were lacking. He looked at me when everything was done, and, teary-eyed, said, "Doc...you kinda saved my life."

HEALTHY GUMS ARE VITAL

It's important for patients to understand that healthy gums – and regular checks to ensure the health of their gums – are vital for oral and overall health. It's also an important prerequisite for just about any cosmetic or dental procedure you want or need to have done. In order to have safe and effective orthodontic treatment, a patient's gums need to be healthy to make sure that the gums can withstand tooth movement. Any type of veneer or crown is also going to involve the gums, so, they need to be in top shape. Healthy, pink gums provide a strong frame for restorative and cosmetic work and ultimately shape how nicely the treatments look once they're done. Also, if the gums aren't healthy, the reality is that the crowns, veneers, and especially implants, can fail, come off, or fall out if the gum tissue recedes or becomes infected, and especially if the bone is affected.

NEW ADVANCEMENTS IN THE TREATMENT OF GUM ISSUES

There have been a host of new advancements when it comes to addressing gum disease and other gum issues. One of the more recent treatments – LANAP – involves using a laser. The LANAP laser enables us to selectively treat diseased areas of the gums without having to open up and move tissue away from the roots of teeth and the jaw bone. The laser is used very precisely around each specific tooth that is impacted. We then can clean the surface of the root so no tartar or calculus builds up. The laser is used, finally, to seal up the pockets around the teeth and ensure that healing can take place.

Tissue engineering and treatment, as I mentioned earlier, is also an advancement. Being able to use donor tissue has become a major benefit and advanced our ability to effectively treat gum issues. We can literally use donor tissue to help patients regrow bone and gum tissue. We also have the ability to add growth factors to the tissue to increase the chance of successful resolution with some of the more complicated cases we treat. For example, if a patient needs an implant, in the past, we'd be forced to place the implant wherever it would fit and had enough bone and gum tissue to support it. Now, with the availability of donor tissue, we can help restore the tissue in the patient's mouth, and then place the implant exactly where it needs to go to be most functional and aesthetically pleasing.

UNTREATED GUM PROBLEMS POSE RISKS

The reasons that gum issues go undiscovered and untreated, sometimes until they pose extreme consequences, vary. Some people are simply afraid of getting dental work done, some are afraid of how bad their oral health may be and so they avoid getting checkups. Sometimes a lack of understanding gum diseases and the risks they pose lead people to neglect or overlook issues they are having. Whatever the reason, it's imperative to understand that neglecting your gums has consequences. The immediate and most obvious risks involve the mouth itself. Gum infections lead to cavities, bone loss, bleeding gums, tooth loss, drainage, and abscesses. More and more research has shown that untreated gum disease and the issues it causes have a direct correlation to the health of the rest of the body as well. Recent studies have shown direct links between gum disease and arthritis, cardiovascular disease, diabetes, Alzheimer's, and cancer.

It's vital, for these reasons, to have regular dental checkups, making sure that the gums are focused on specifically to check for early signs of problems and to help establish treatment plans that will curb any problems that are found during checkups. Gingivitis, with regular professional maintenance and proper home care, is entirely reversible. Periodontitis, while not reversible, is treatable, as I've discussed above. Remember that, whatever the state of your oral health, if it's addressed as early as possible, it can be treated and you can salvage your teeth and your smile.

KNOW THE SIGNS

One of the best ways to treat gum disease and other oral health issues is to know the early signs or indicators that there might be a problem. One of the first things patients often notice, especially with gingivitis, is that when they brush or floss, their spit looks pink. This is an indication that the gums are bleeding. Sometimes patients actually see blood in their mouth. This is a good indication that gum disease is brewing.

Pain also accompanies this. Sometimes it's pain related to the brushing and flossing that causes the bleeding. Pain in the form of sensitivity to hot and cold foods and drinks – as I mentioned earlier – is also an indicator that there are some gum problems that need to be addressed. Other indicators that patients commonly talk about are bad breath, noticing gaping or spaces forming between teeth, loose teeth, and obvious gum recession.

COSTS

It's difficult to put specific price points on treatments for gum problems because it will, of course, vary depending on the region of the country you get treatment in, the doctor that you see, and what type of insurance plan you have. Unfortunately, most dental plans don't believe that there is any significant functionality benefit for treating gummy smiles, so there often isn't a lot of coverage for those. In my practice, we always write narratives for each case. To give some examples so that you have a better idea of price ranges you might be looking at for some procedures, I can say that to do a crown lengthening treatment for a gummy smile which treats four to six teeth, you'll be looking at a cost of somewhere between $2,000 and $3,000. For treatments like the grafting procedures we do, my practice doesn't charge extra for the use of donor tissue, however, some practices might. Depending on how many teeth we need to address, a patient would be looking at anywhere from $1,500 up to $3,000. The pinhole procedure we do also runs around the same price range.

THE RELUCTANT PROFESSIONAL

I'd like to share one more story. This patient's journey is different than most because she didn't really understand why she was sent to see me and had no idea how profoundly her life could be changed.

This patient, a woman in her early sixties, is a medical professional. She knows a lot about the body and the skin. She was incredibly reluctant when she first came to see me. She'd been to see her general dentist and was prepared to do six crowns in the front of her mouth. She did, however, have a very gummy smile and her dentist referred her to me.

She told me the first time I met her, "I don't really understand why I'm here. I just want to get my crowns done. I don't really think there's anything wrong with my smile." That's when I took her through the issues that I saw with her gums and showed her what could be done to correct it, making her crowns, ultimately, look better and be more sustainable in the long run.

We ended up doing a crown lengthening procedure, reducing the amount of gum tissue. Even after this was done, she still wasn't entirely convinced that it had been necessary. The real change came when she finally got her crowns put in. I'm willing to bet that no one had ever seen this lady smile as largely and as proudly as she did once her crowns were installed. She saw the immediate and drastic difference that the crown lengthening procedure had made with the final result. The biggest hurdle was really that she didn't realize what an aesthetic difference could be made by treating her gummy smile before she received her crowns. She'd just accepted her gummy smile as being the best that she could hope for. It was a wonderful experience to be able to offer her an even more beautiful smile than she'd even considered was possible. To this day, she is so happy with her treatment that she proudly tells anyone who will listen about her smile transformation.

This story also brings to light one thing that I'd like all patients to keep in mind. Ask for options. When you're talking to your dentist, periodontist, orthodontist – whoever – feel free to ask what options are available to give you the very best outcome, aesthetically and in overall health. If you're comfortable with your smile, it's still okay to be educated about the possibilities that are out there, treatments that could transform the way you look, feel, and function. Being informed before you make decisions about your treatment is a critical piece of the puzzle that I think all patients should be embracing. It never hurts to have all the facts. And, as this patient's story reveals, exposing yourself to the variety of options available could just transform your smile and your life.

ABOUT JESSICA STILLEY, DMD, MS

Periodontal Health Center
www.periodontalhealthcenter.com

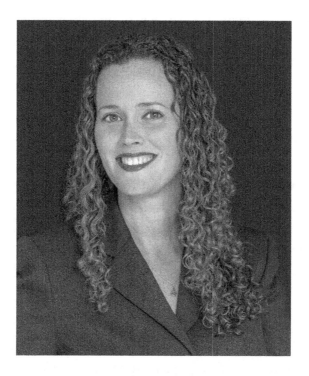

Dr. Jessica Stilley is a Tampa Bay Area dentist with a focus on periodontal disease prevention and treatment. Dr. Stilley received her DMD from the University of Florida in 2005 and obtained a Master's degree in Oral Biology as well as a Certificate in Periodontics from The Ohio State University in 2008. She is trained in traditional periodontal therapy as well as LANAP, Pinhole technique and implant placement and site preparation.

Along with her credentials and training, Dr. Stilley has collected numerous accolades and awards. She is currently a Line Officer on the Executive Council of the West Coast District Dental Association and the Executive Council of the Florida Association of Periodontists. She is an Anesthesia Inspector for the Florida Board of Dentistry and was Past President of the West Pasco Dental Association.

Dr. Stilley is fluent in Spanish and English, helping patients to understand their treatment and seek the best options for periodontal and dental care. She is also a member of the American Dental Association, the American Academy of Periodontology, and the American Dental Society of Anesthesiology.

Dr. Stilley is passionate about the fight to prevent and treat periodontal disease, and works with patients every day to ensure that they do not lose their teeth due to gum issues. She focuses on periodontal treatment as well as other types of preventative dentistry and offers IV sedation for many procedures. Dr. Stilley and her team are dedicated to helping patients avoid tooth loss caused by periodontal disease by working with them to identify and treat gum problems in the early stages.

Dr. Stilley and her team offer both periodontal pocket reduction and regeneration surgery as well as plastic surgery and reconstruction. Dr. Stilley also offers pre-implant surgery and implant therapy, periodontal surgery for orthodontics, and periodontal maintenance. Along with her team, Dr. Stilley offers patients sedation and treatment options to ensure that they receive the most comfortable care possible. She routinely helps patients with serious gum disease issues and finds solutions to create a beautiful, healthy smile that will last a lifetime.

SMILE MAKEOVER WITH PORCELAIN VENEERS

A great smile is something that everyone would love. Often, patients have structural issues that can cause a host of symptoms, the least of which is a less-than-ideal smile. When the issue is purely appearance related, veneers are a highly effective treatment option for many patients, one that can provide a perfect smile. However, it is not just about appearance. The reality is that a person with an aesthetically displeasing smile is usually affected on a deeper emotional and psychological level, such as in their interactions with others and how they ultimately feel about themselves. My goal is to provide every patient with the very best care and with a smile that they can be proud to show off.

VENEERS AND THEIR PURPOSE

A veneer is a porcelain shell that is bonded over the front and edges of a tooth. The most common use of veneers is to alleviate visible flaws on a patient's teeth. In many cases, patients choose veneers because they are not satisfied with the color or shape of their teeth. Patients may also desire to correct gaps between teeth or repair partially cracked or chipped teeth. Veneers can be used for patients who feel that their teeth look either too short or too long. We can adjust the original teeth and apply veneers to correct that issue. Veneers are an amazing, versatile restorative option used in cosmetic dentistry today.

Many patients consider veneers to remedy cracked, chipped, or worn-down teeth. Depending on the severity of the damage and what caused it, veneers may be the ideal option. For example, if someone has been in an accident that resulted in chipped or fractured teeth, veneers can be a great option. However, if the teeth have extensive decay and are severely broken down, or if the patient has a systemic condition or infection that is affecting their oral health, then those underlying issues need to be addressed before considering veneers.

Another reason veneers are such a great restorative option is because they are one of the most conservative cosmetic treatments available and they provide an almost instantaneous change in the way their teeth and smile look. If a patient has, for example, crowding or gaps between their teeth, or a portion of a tooth has fractured, a dentist can correct these issues with veneers in a matter of just two or three visits.

WHAT VENEERS CAN DO FOR YOU

To better illustrate the positive impact veneers can have, I'd like to share a story with you about one of my patients.

Eve was very self-conscious about her smile when she came to see me. She shared that, in her younger years, she was sick a lot and that she was prescribed the antibiotic tetracycline. This antibiotic was used fairly commonly in the 1950's and 1960's for a variety of illnesses in children. However, it became clear, over time, that one of the major side effects of the drug was the gray and brown bands it caused to form on the developing adult teeth. Eve spent her entire childhood, teenage life, and up through her forties feeling ashamed of her smile, which was severely impacted by the excessive amount of tetracycline she had taken as a child.

She was treated by her former dentist approximately a decade before coming to my office. This dentist tried to utilize bonding to mask the extensive discolorations of her teeth, but the bonding was in no way effective in improving the esthetics of her smile. After evaluating the condition of her teeth in my office, we discussed treatment options, and eventually, decided she would benefit greatly from the placement of 10 veneers. At 56 years old, Eve looked at the results and told me, with tears in her eyes, "For the first time in my life, I have a beautiful smile!"

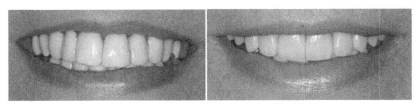

Before and after placing veneers (Eve)

If nothing else, this patient's story illustrates just how successful and life-changing veneers can be in terms of correcting cosmetic damage, improving a patient's appearance, and also improving their self-image, self-confidence and how they feel about themselves. When you are able to drastically improve someone's appearance by giving them a genuinely beautiful smile, you can not only see the difference, but you can *feel* the difference it makes in their life.

TYPES OF VENEERS

Porcelain veneers are created using different grades of porcelain, but their exact construction and look varies greatly based on the brand. Some of the more common brands I utilize in my cases to help achieve beautiful, natural results are Emax,

Empress and Da Vinci veneers. Some brands are stronger, but maybe aren't quite as aesthetically pleasing, and some are more esthetic, but not quite as strong or durable.

Each patient is assessed individually to determine which veneer will work best for their lifestyle and the look they want. Then, I discuss the various options available to them, and develop a treatment plan that will move them towards their goal. In the case of patients who tend to clench and grind their teeth, or who engage in sports or other activities that may put extra pressure on their teeth, I will urge them to use a night guard or sports guard for protection, just as I would for a patient with natural teeth.

RECONTOURING TEETH FOR VENEERS

The amount of recontouring of the teeth required before veneers can be applied varies for each individual patient and situation. Prior to beginning any case, I fabricate diagnostic study models and take photographs of the patient's teeth. These diagnostic tools are then shared with the talented lab technicians that I work with and together we design the final look of the veneers. The lab technician prepares a "wax up" of the case which is a wax model of the proposed final veneers. The technicians fabricate a preparation guide with information that helps me determine the type of recontouring the patient needs to aid with the design of the veneers. I utilize this guide, along with the wax model, to ensure that the teeth are properly designed and that the patient achieves the smile they desire.

The veneer design is always customized for each individual and the goal is to be as conservative as possible. Generally, I try to keep veneers about the thickness of a fingernail – no thicker than that. For the veneers to fit properly and look flawless, it is necessary to recontoure enough of the patient's underlying teeth to accommodate the thickness of the veneers.

In cases where the recontouring needs to be a little more extensive, slightly more of the tooth might need to be adjusted, and the veneer would be made a little thicker to account for this. For example, if a patient has teeth that are heavily discolored, and they are looking for a bright, white smile, then the recontouring for veneers would need to be a bit more extensive. Since the porcelain material is essentially glass, the shade of the teeth under the veneers will impact the final color and, ultimately, the esthetics of the case.

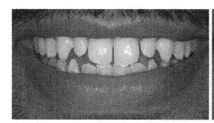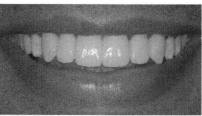

Before and after placing veneers

Veneers are bonded to the teeth by the dentist using a special cement. The bonding process is strengthened by first "conditioning" the tooth with a conditioning gel. This gel creates a rougher surface texture which increases the bond of the veneer to the tooth. Bonding veneers is usually a very straightforward process, and patients on occasion will not require anesthetic for the application procedure. Once the veneers are in place, the dentist checks them for fit, shape, and color, and makes any necessary adjustments.

PREPLESS VENEERS

Prepless veneers are a different veneer option and, as their name suggests, do not require any recontouring of the teeth before they are applied. This means that the dentist does not need to modify the patient's teeth before the veneers are put on but this technique is only used in very specific situations.

The patients who are usually a good fit for prepless veneers are those with small teeth, or with gaps or unfilled spaces in between the teeth. In these cases, prepless veneers are used to fill in the missing volume and make up for the lack in size of their natural teeth.

ADVANTAGES OF VENEERS VS. TEETH WHITENING TREATMENTS

Veneers offer patients a superior cosmetic alternative to traditional teeth whitening treatments. With whitening treatments, the results are uncontrolled and can vary significantly, even from one tooth in an arch to the tooth right beside it. Basically, the result is, "You get whatever you get". The end result can leave a patient with some teeth coming out very, very white – the way the patient wants all their teeth to look – and with others that are not so very bright and white. That is especially true with "at home" whitening kits that are sold over-the-counter. A more dramatic, consistent result is achieved with a professional "in office" whitening treatment from a dentist.

If a patient has previous dental restorations – for example crowns, fillings, or veneers, traditional whitening treatments will not change the color of those restorations. It is only effective on natural teeth. Also, a whitening treatment, of course, doesn't address other possible issues that a patient may want to take care of, such as worn down, chipped or broken teeth, gaps in between teeth, or slightly crowded, rotated, or misaligned teeth. With veneers, a dentist can address any or all of these issues, while creating a beautiful, bright white smile.

As far as color or shade of teeth, with veneers, we can get the exact color the patient desires, because – unlike traditional whitening treatments – we can control it. For a skilled dentist and lab technician, veneers make it very straightforward to give patients exactly the shade of whiteness and level of brightness they desire. If they have existing restorations, such as a crown or fillings, the dentist can change the crown to match the color of the veneers since the porcelain used to fabricate veneers is the same porcelain that is used to fabricate crowns.

And finally, veneers are a long lasting restoration, while traditional tooth whitening is just a temporary treatment measure and, in fact, there's really no way to predict how long the whitening will last. How long a whitening treatment lasts depends on many different factors – things like diet, smoking and the quality of attention given to day-to-day dental hygiene practices. For example, if a patient drinks a lot of coffee or wine, or smokes, their teeth are going to stain and lose that whiteness a lot faster. Porcelain veneers, on the other hand, resist staining from things such as coffee, wine or smoking.

ADVANTAGES OF VENEERS VS. TRADITIONAL ORTHODONTIC TREATMENT

Veneers offer great advantages over traditional orthodontic treatment. In cases where a patient has large gaps between their teeth – or the opposite problem, slightly crowded teeth – we may be able to use veneers to resolve those issues and give the patient a life-changing new smile in just a couple of visits. Think about what a huge advantage that is for the patient, as compared to having to go through orthodontic treatment that could take up to a year or maybe even longer.

It is not just the time involved, although of course being able to take care of everything in just one or two visits is a huge benefit. Many patients hesitate to embark on the long, drawn-out process of orthodontics. Having important life events such as weddings, birthdays or starting a new job, may concerns patients with regard to being photographed while stuck in the middle of orthodontics. Once the orthodontic treatment process is finally completed, the patient will have to wear retainers for the rest of their life, in order to keep the teeth straight. Once the teeth are moved into the ideal position, retainers keep the teeth from shifting back to their original position.

With veneers, there are no retainers needed because the teeth have not been moved. Patients give huge sighs of relief and big, grateful smiles ponce they understand there is an option other orthodontics and that their case can be completed with veneers in just a couple of visits. They brighten up immediately when they realize they can have the beautiful smile they desire in the next *couple of weeks,* instead of the in the next *year.*

USING VENEERS WITH OTHER DENTAL TREATMENT THERAPIES

While veneers can be utilized to address a variety of cosmetic dental issues on their own, they can also be paired with other dental treatment options to offer a comprehensive cosmetic result. A patient may require the restoration of multiple teeth, for example, a combination of porcelain crowns and veneers. The boutique dental labs I work with are able to achieve a perfect color match for crowns and the veneers, and no one will know the difference – no one looking at your teeth will be able to tell which restorations are crowns and which are the veneers. They will all have a brilliant, life-like appearance!

I also highly recommend that patients have professional teeth whitening prior to starting a veneer case. This will allow me to ensure that the teeth are as bright as possible before we choose a color for the finished veneers.

While it is more common to do veneers on the upper teeth because they show most prominently when smiling or in photos, patients still desire to have an appealing, match in appearance between the upper and lower teeth. The solution? Porcelain veneers on the upper teeth and then use a professional whitening treatment on the lower teeth to even out the esthetics of the arches.

Many patients require a case that uses varied treatment modalities in different phases to create the desired end result. For instance, a patient with very badly misaligned teeth might not initially be a good candidate for veneers. Traditional orthodontic treatment or Invisalign® may be the best treatment option for correcting severe misalignment or a bad bite. Then, once the orthodontic treatment is complete, the patient can proceed with veneers to take care of the remaining cosmetic concerns. In steps, I can give a patient the "Movie Star" smile they've always wanted.

THE COST OF VENEERS

The price of veneers varies greatly and can depend on many factors. The geographic area where they have them done, the clinical skill level of the doctor, the type and number of veneers, the skill and reputation of the lab that creates them, and even why they are getting the veneers. Dental insurance usually doesn't cover veneers because it's largely a cosmetic procedure. In my experience, working in the northeast – New York and New Jersey – I have seen veneers range from $1,200 up to $2,500 in places like New York City.

A lot of the cost depends on the number of veneers a patient gets and the complexity of the case. Most patients do not come in for only one or two veneers. In many cases, you might, in the long run, end up paying more if you try to get by with fewer veneers than you really need. When I assess each patient, I ask them to smile, take photos and models of their teeth, evaluate their bite and address whatever concerns the patients has and then I recommend the number of veneers based on this information.

To use an analogy, the price variation is somewhat like the varying prices you might pay for a new car. The price tag depends a lot on what type of car you're buying, the size of the engine, any additional features that come with the car and, of course, the reputation of the car company. You wouldn't expect to get a top of the line Mercedes or Lamborghini for the same price as a basic Toyota. Basically, you get what you pay for in terms of both quality and aesthetics.

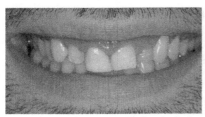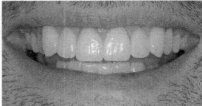

Before and after placing veneers

Do Your Research before Getting Veneers

I think it goes without saying that it's important for you, as a patient, to know about and understand veneers, and more importantly, to be informed about the doctor making and placing the veneers.

There are some common misconceptions that people have about veneers. Some people think they may look fake or phony.

Patients have used the word "Chicklet" to describe veneers that look big or bulky. Chicklets were a brand of gum that came in the form of large, white, candy squares. And veneers – if they're <u>not</u> done right, by a skilled dentist – can have that sort of big or bulky appearance. But if veneers are done properly, you're not going to have that problem.

Another misconception is that some people think that their teeth are going to be irreversibly damaged from a veneer. In reality, a veneer is actually the most conservative tooth preparation that a dentist can do. I explain to patients that most veneers are usually no more than the thickness of a fingernail. Veneers are a very conservative treatment option in terms of dental restorations.

Some people may have seen photos on the internet or heard horror stories about how unnatural veneers can look. This only reinforces how important it is for patients to do their research and find a dentist who is well-trained and experienced in the art of applying veneers. Before you let a dentist treat you, be sure to ask to see before and after photos of cases they have completed personally, that are similar to yours.

To do veneers properly, a dentist needs the proper training and practice. I encourage every patient considering veneers to do their homework and find out what type of training and experience a dentist has in relation to veneers. How long have they been practicing? What type of education and training have they received? How many cases have they treated with veneers? What is the success rate of the veneers they've placed? These are all important questions to have answered before you let a doctor treat you. A credible and reputable dentist should have no problem answering all of these questions, and any other questions or concerns you may have.

I have been in practice since 1996 and I am committed to continually advancing my dental knowledge and education. I constantly seek out the top doctors and dentists in different techniques and glean knowledge from them. I pursue seminars, workshops, conferences, and opportunities to learn more from the very best practitioners. Most states only require about 30 to 40 educational credits every few years to maintain your dental license. I attend classes worth hundreds of credits every single year because I am eager to advance my skills and have the most up-to-date knowledge on every aspect of cosmetic dentistry, especially when it comes to veneers. I am committed to giving my patients the very best experience and getting the very best results.

THE LIFE-CHANGING EFFECTS OF A GREAT SMILE

People do not feel good about themselves when they are uncomfortable with their smile. Constantly hiding or covering your smile, or avoiding smiling altogether, can lead to individuals becoming depressed, disillusioned, and dissatisfied with themselves. It affects how they are treated and how they treat others. To illustrate this point, I'd like to share one final story with you.

Cheryl, a lovely lady in her mid to late 40s, came to see me not that long ago. She didn't smile much. She brought a bunch of pictures with her and showed them to me. These were family portraits of her and her siblings. "Do you see the commonality in my photos?" I wasn't sure what she was referring to. "See how beautiful my siblings' teeth are? I never smile in photos." It was then I noticed that in all of her pictures, Cheryl definitely wasn't smiling. She was very embarrassed by her teeth. I could see the long-reaching effects of this on her face and in her demeanor. "When I'm done with you, you won't be able to stop smiling," I told her. Then, we did a huge smile makeover using beautiful veneers. When I see her now, she can't help but smile. She tells me and shows me how proudly she smiles in all pictures now. Cheryl's smile is now on par with, or perhaps even better than, that of her siblings.

The joy and pride that a patient feels with a brand-new smile always resonates with me. This is why I love what I do and always strive to give my patients my very best. Yes, veneers are cosmetic. But adjusting an aspect of a patient's physical appearance that they're unhappy with – being able to give them the look they desire - is something that affects their whole life, not just the way they look. I'm able to offer my patients more than just beautiful teeth. Veneers offer a great smile, and that transformation is often totally life-changing.

About Todd Goldstein, DDS

NJ Laser Dentistry
www.njlaserdentistry.com
The Exchange Dental Group
www.theexchangedentalgroup.com

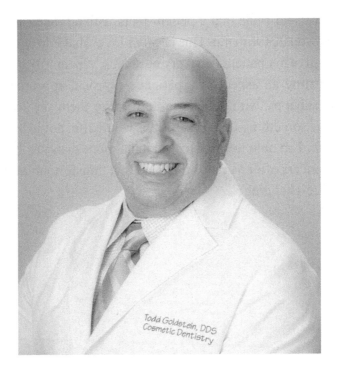

Dr. Todd Goldstein received his B.S. In Biology from The University at Stonybrook and his D.D.S. from University at Buffalo School of Dental Medicine. After graduation in 1996, Dr. Goldstein completed a one year general practice residency at Maimonides Medical Center in Brooklyn, NY. Since then, Dr. Goldstein has completed thousands of hours in advanced continuing education. His emphasis of study has been in the restoration of health, dental aesthetics and function to people with compromised or missing teeth. The intensive training and knowledge that Dr. Goldstein brings to his practice leads to longer, happier and healthier lives for his patients.

Dr. Goldstein also has specialized training in cosmetic, restorative and implant dentistry and holds or has held memberships in several distinctive dental societies including the American Dental Association, New Jersey Dental Association, Academy of General Dentistry, American Academy of Cosmetic Dentistry and the International Congress of Oral Implantology where he received fellowship status. Dr. Goldstein is also certified in the placement of invisible orthodontic aligners using Invisalign® and Clear Correct.

When not in the office Dr. Goldstein loves spending his free time with his wife Karina, and his sons Alex and Tyler. He also enjoys exercising, reading and is an avid sports enthusiast.

BITING RIGHT IS LIVING RIGHT

Having a great smile is about much more than just proper alignment and beautiful teeth. On a much deeper level, having a great smile is vital because of the way it affects a person's self-image, how they project themselves and how they feel as individuals. There are a variety of things that can affect a person's confidence in their smile. Temporomandibular joint disorder, otherwise known in my profession as TMD, is just one.

In the briefest sense, TMD is any disordered state of the temporomandibular joint that affects the way a person's jaw and mouth functions.

THE IMPORTANCE OF HAVING A GOOD BITE

Before I share one example of a case I worked on, I'd like to talk briefly about what constitutes a good bite. To keep it simple, a good bite involves the top and bottom teeth, especially the back teeth, lining up in such a way that the muscles of the jaw and the jaw joints remain in a comfortable, relaxed state when the teeth connect. For this to happen, the upper and lower jaws need to be in proper alignment.

A good bite is important for many reasons, but it's easiest to identify these by looking at the consequences of NOT having a good bite. When a patient's teeth don't line up properly, the muscles that control jaw movements become strained and are forced to work harder to compensate for the lack of alignment. Every time the patient chews, swallows, or speaks – things which occur roughly 3,000 times per day – the muscles experience strain in order to allow the teeth to come together. As a result, we often see patients with constant headaches, jaw pain, neck pain, back pain, and even ear pain and ringing in the ears. While there are a whole host of other problems misalignment of the jaw can cause, these tend to be the most common.

ONE OF MY EARLIEST CASES

I'd like to offer one of the earliest cases I worked on as a good example of exactly what TMD can look like and the issues it can cause.

Early in my career, I had a nurse referred to me by a local pain management doctor who had been treating her for severe pain caused by something known as trigeminal neuralgia, an extremely painful neurological disorder. The pain management doctor had been treating this woman with very powerful painkillers and occasional injections in her head in an attempt to relieve her excruciating pain. Having to constantly take painkillers was having a noticeable and significantly negative effect on her quality of life. She wasn't herself. She had difficulty functioning, couldn't drive, and eventually was unable to continue working.

This course of treatment, despite the drastic effects on her life, was having limited success in treating her pain. The trigeminal nerve, which is split, runs through both halves of the brain.

Because this was the nerve causing her debilitating pain, she ended up having brain surgery on one half of her head to help take some of the pressure off.

When she was referred to me, she'd had this surgery and was planning for an operation on the other half of her brain because her pain still persisted. I attended a conference with her pain management doctor and he told me about her case, and that he thought she might have some temporomandibular joint issues. He also thought those issues might be the cause of some of her pain and that I might be able to help. After examining her and taking a close look at her case, I realized that most of her trigeminal neuralgia pain was being caused by an extremely bad bite that was indeed the result of TMD issues.

The nurse's case involved a variety of treatments and it was a long road to resolution. But in the end, she was a new woman. She returned to work, started driving again, and returned to her normal life. One of the best outcomes of the treatment was the fact that she didn't have to have the second brain surgery. Together with her other physicians, we were able to cut the severe pain out of her life. This, more than anything, allowed her to smile with confidence, and with a truly beautiful smile. To this day, her story is one I hold close to my heart.

WHAT IS TMD?

Again, TMD is a disorder of the temporomandibular joint. When talking about this issue, it's usually shortened to just TMJ or TMD (temporomandibular disorder). We all have temporomandibular joints on each side of our head, joints that attach to the lower jaw, otherwise known as the mandible. A disorder of these joints also involves the complex system of muscles that control the movements of our jaws.

These two joints are the only two in the entire body that are connected to one bone, meaning they have to work harmoniously for the jaw to function properly. TMD means that the joints are not working together for one or more reasons. There is a wide array of symptoms with TMD. As I mentioned earlier, jaw pain, headaches, neck and back pain are all common symptoms. Other symptoms include things that wouldn't seem to be related to the jaw at all, things such as numbness of the fingers, cold hands, and cold feet. This is just a brief sprinkling of the symptoms involved with this disorder - there are dozens of other possible symptoms that can be associated with TMD.

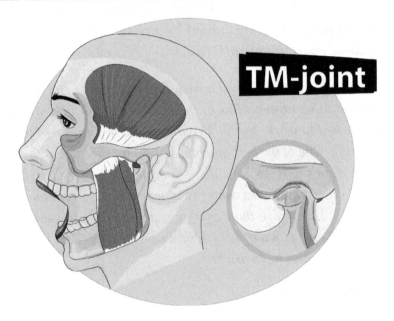

It's easy to see how one's quality of life can be profoundly affected by TMD. Our most basic survival needs – breathing, eating, and swallowing – depend on a properly functioning jaw. So when TMD disrupts our ability to perform these most basic and necessary functions, it impacts so much more than our smile. The deficit the disorder can cause in the functioning of the temporomandibular joints causes imbalance and stress within the entire body's system that can have far-reaching effects. This includes impacting your sleep, your ability to work, and your overall nutrition because more nutritious foods are generally more difficult to chew, something that is usually avoided by people with TMD.

THE VISUALS OF TMD

After treating patients with TMD for a number of years now, one of the most striking things I've noticed is the facial features that many patients have in common, especially in the mid-face region. For example, it's not uncommon to see that patients suffering from TMD seem to have less space between their nose and their chin, often leading them to look older. Also, many patients with the disorder tend to have a recessed chin, a chin that's set back so as to give the appearance of an overbite, whether they actually have one or not. This goes a long way in affecting the person's profile and the general overall balance and aesthetics of their face. Sometimes, they have what we would call a flat or dished-in face, again because the jaws don't function properly.

This isn't the case for all individuals suffering from TMD, however, it's common enough that they are markers or signs that I look for when trying to determine whether TMD might be the culprit causing whatever symptoms they're having.

The other major issue when it comes to aesthetics is actually a result of the problem with pain that most TMD sufferers experience. Often, any type of movement with the mouth and jaw, especially smiling, causes at least some pain or discomfort for the patient. This often leads to patients having a distorted, asymmetric smile that is uneven. This asymmetry, conjoined with the overworking of the jaw muscles, and unevenness of the working of the jaw muscles, tends to leave patients with a facial appearance that stands out in an unflattering way.

FIXING A BAD BITE

In my business, fixing a bad bite – known as malocclusion – is always important when patients need extensive dental treatment. Also, I should note that almost everyone has at least a little bit of malocclusion, and so having a bad bite doesn't necessarily mean the person suffers from TMD. Untreated TMD oftentimes results in breakdown of healthy teeth over time.

One of the first things I do with every patient is to take frontal and profile photos, as well as pictures of their teeth. Using these pictures, I initially work up an analysis of their case in terms of what they need to have done and how extensive a treatment plan I need to set up. When dealing with a bad bite, I look for things like gum recession, gum line notches, and indentations in the teeth. These are all strong signs that there is a loss of stability in their bite, whether with one or a few teeth, or with the whole mouth. In the past, before there was a good understanding of TMD, dentists used to sometimes tell their patients that they were brushing too hard and that that was causing the recession. In reality, brushing has nothing to do with it. It's all about the forces on the teeth and in the jaw and how it's all distributed.

After doing the photos for the initial workup, I'll start to ask a patient questions about common TMD symptoms like popping, clicking, headaches, and other pain. Unless these symptoms are severe, prolonged, or pointed out to them, some patients may not even realize they have significant bite problems and therefore may not do anything to correct them.

Treatment-wise, there are a number of approaches to correcting a bad bite. If it's very obvious that one or several teeth are the culprits, these can be addressed on a specific basis. If, for example, it's clear that one tooth is too tall or out of position, I might be able to trim that tooth or apply a treatment to straighten the tooth, and fix the bite problem with minimal work. If more than one tooth is involved, I have a special electronic sensor I use which measures the force balance in the mouth and reveals which teeth are being impacted and by how much. I can use this to perform a coronoplasty, or bite equilibration, where I contour and reshape the teeth and even out the bite that way. While this isn't my favorite way of dealing with bite issues, it's relatively quick and painless for the patient and usually provides good results.

If the teeth are generally in good condition with not much wear and not a lot of existing dental work, but the bite is considerably off, the best solution may be neuromuscular (also called physiologic) orthodontic treatment. What makes this approach different than traditional orthodontics is that the primary focus is on finding a comfortable jaw position for the jaw joints and the muscles, and once that's confirmed, to then move the teeth to support and maintain this position long term. This type of treatment requires advanced training, so be sure to do your research on who can provide this type of service.

Another type of orthodontic treatment that I provide for less complicated bite cases is invisalign® clear aligners. These move a patient's teeth that are absorbing more force or pressure than they can handle. This is a very successful way to adjust a bad bite. What's nice about Invisalign® is that as the name implies, it's nearly invisible, and it's more comfortable because the aligners can be removed for eating and brushing teeth.

None of these methods, of course, treat recession of gums or teeth, so, once I've addressed the bad bite, those types of issues would still need to be addressed with further treatment. However, correcting the bite will at least prevent further damage and is an important step in restoring good overall oral health for the patient.

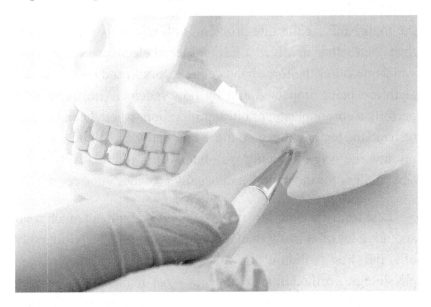

TREATING TMD

The simple fact is that there isn't one simple answer to the question of how to treat patients with TMD, because every case is different and every patient has different symptoms or combination of symptoms that affect what types of treatments will work best.

First, it's important to determine through objective diagnostic testing where each patient is, what their baseline condition is, what symptoms they have, and how their neuromuscular system is functioning. The neuromuscular system, to reiterate, controls the nerves and muscles of the head, neck, and jaw, and how each area functions, both individually and together. Once this information has been gathered, a dentist utilizes a CT scanner to determine the alignment of a patient's jaw joints. It shows exactly how the joints are lining up and also offers us a lot of information about obstructions to a patient's airway that may exist because of the alignment.

All of this information then must be reviewed by the dentist to determine if the patient is neuromuscularly stable. If they are not, pertinent background information about potential causes for the instability should be investigated, like whether the patient fell or was in an accident. This helps the dentist determine if there might be structural damage to the joints, if there's a bone problem, or if there's damage to the muscles. In order to effectively treat the patient, the dentist needs to know if there's a bone issue or joint issue, a muscle issue, or a combination of these.

Treating TMD is typically unlike general dentistry because it's not as straightforward. We have set procedures and treatments for things like cavities, gum disease, and decayed teeth. Treating the TMJ is much more complex and generally requires a great deal more patience and time. In many of the cases I've treated, longstanding TMJ damage has occurred because of a lack of noticeable symptoms. Damage that has been there for years, that has occurred over time and been left untreated, can't ever be truly repaired in the sense that I can't go back and reverse the damage. I can't take a damaged joint and return it to its original, healthy condition, much as I wish I could. My end goal is to contain the damage, manage the symptoms, and prevent any further deterioration or disruption of the joint and surrounding tissues.

RECOVERING FROM TMD

The amount of time it takes a patient to recover from TMD, with treatment, really depends primarily on how much time has elapsed since the onset of their symptoms as well as their age. As with any disease, the earlier the problem is diagnosed, the better the chances are of lessening the overall damage and thus cutting down on the amount of time it takes to see positive results from treatment and get the patient into recovery.

In order to discuss recovery, we have to go back to the fact that TMD has such a broad spectrum of symptoms, many that can be disregarded by patients or misdiagnosed as other things. Many of the symptoms often mask the underlying TMD. I've actually lost count, unfortunately, of the number of patients I've treated for TMD who were initially treated incorrectly for a whole host of other issues. The list is long, but a lot of the common misdiagnoses include ear infections, chronic migraines, allergies, and sinus infections. This, unfortunately, means that patients can go for years with TMJ-related pain that is undiagnosed TMD. In such cases, they are ultimately much slower to recover due to the extensive amount of wear and tear on the joints and the damage that has already occurred.

As I mentioned, age plays a major factor in recovery time as well. As is true with most treatments, the younger the patient, the quicker they usually are to respond to treatment and the faster they are to heal and recover. However, because the issues I just discussed regarding misdiagnosis or TMD going unnoticed for longer and longer periods of time, the majority of the patients I treat for TMD are adults, with the average age being somewhere in the 40s or 50s. These patients have often suffered from the effects of TMD for far too long, and that means that it takes them longer to recover. More education on TMD and other TMJ issues, along with the ease of access to the information because of the internet, has led to more and more people recognizing they need to be checked for possible TMD, if for no other reason than to rule it out. Still, with most of the patients I see, significant damage has been done to the joints before the patient come to be treated.

Regardless, I treat every patient according to their unique needs. I give them hope that we can do something to treat their symptoms, get their pain under control, and keep the disease from doing any more damage. There's always something that can be done to help them.

In terms of starting recovery through treatment, I would say that treatment for TMD usually takes between six and eight weeks to truly start seeing results. Some patients notice a major difference very early in the treatment process, while others may take a little longer. Ultimately, just as treatment is very individualized, the speed and amount of recovery made at every stage of treatment are also unique to the patient.

THE FINANCIAL COST OF TREATING TMD

This question gets brought up a lot because, unfortunately, most dental insurances – and medical, as well – don't cover TMD treatment, and if it does at all, they don't usually cover the entire cost. My practice has found, however, that as we treat more and more cases of TMD and have successful results, we are seeing more reimbursement from different medical plans. Regardless, it shouldn't be relied upon. Think of it as a gift if insurance does cover some of the expense.

To give a conservative estimate, I'd say that treating TMD, on average, costs somewhere in the $4,000 to $7,000 range. This will vary, of course, by provider and the area of the country you're in. In my experience, it takes about three months for an effective treatment plan to be developed and executed, and most practitioners treating TMD would allow this same amount of time. This means that the fee I quoted above should roughly cover a three-month period of treatment, including time for the workup, treatment, and recovery.

Preventing a Bad Bite

Of course, the best way to treat a bad bite and/or TMD is to prevent it in the first place or catch it as soon as possible. Preventing tooth decay and damage goes a really long way to accomplishing both of these goals. Maintaining the strength of your teeth – and thereby your bite – is key. Tooth loss, aside from having wisdom teeth removed, can have long-term detrimental effects on the stability of your bite and your joints.

Keep up regular checkups with your dentist. This is crucial for your overall health, especially the health of your mouth, teeth, and gums. Even if you're not having any particular issues, it's a good idea to see your regular dentist at least once every six months. This allows you to have at least two really good, professional, thorough cleanings twice a year and makes it easier to catch any issues with your teeth and your bite early on and quickly prevent them from getting any worse.

More on Preventing TMD

Unfortunately, there isn't a massive amount that can be done to prevent TMD and damage if you are susceptible to joint conditions or if the condition has gone untreated for some time. This leads back to what I mentioned earlier – the key to stopping TMD and the damage it wreaks on your jaw and ultimately your entire body is to get the disease diagnosed and treated as early as possible. Seeing your dentist regularly can help with this.

Many general dentists can't or don't treat TMD, however, most are very good at recognizing potential signs of the disease and can refer you to a doctor who can offer treatment. Some key symptoms to watch for are clicking and/or popping when you talk, chew, yawn, or otherwise move your jaw. Also, pain, such as recurring headaches or earaches are common indications that there might be something going on with your TMJ. Even if these symptoms don't seem particularly troubling to you, mention them to your dentist. The dentist can check your teeth, your bite, and other basic structural issues and help to determine if you should seek further evaluation.

ASK QUESTIONS

I get a lot of common questions from patients that I treat for TMD. They want to know why they were fine a few months ago and are suddenly having issues and pain. The best way I can explain this is to offer an analogy. I encourage my patients to think about TMD as a bucket that gets water poured into it. TMD is not generally an acute disorder, but rather something that builds up over time. I tell my patients to think about a bucket that constantly gets different portions of water dumped into it over time. Eventually, the bucket becomes full and overflows. That overflow is the shift in symptoms they experience.

I encourage anyone being treated for TMD – or really any dental treatment – to ask questions. Be involved in your own treatment. The best way I have to treat you successfully is to know what questions and concerns you have and answer them. This process of question and answer also provides me with a lot of the details I need to know about what's been bothering you, and what symptoms you're experiencing that I can't see or hear. A lot of times, the photos I take during the evaluation stage, as well as progress photos and scans I take during the process of treatment, are great tools to answer my patient's questions. I can show you directly what's going on in your jaw and head, and give you a visual that may answer many of the questions you have.

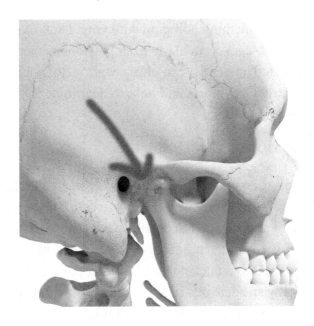

ONE FINAL STORY

To really encapsulate everything I've written here, and to give you a better idea of why I do what I do, I'd like to share one final story.

This case is one of my most recent cases. A patient came to see me after developing severe vertigo, dizziness, and loss of balance. The patient's vertigo had started two years previous and she'd seen a number of specialists. No one could put their finger on exactly what was causing it. She had an MRI done and numerous brain scans to check for tumors. Doctors looked at her to see if she had sinus or ear issues that might be the cause. She also saw a litany of therapists, both physical and massage therapists. Regardless of whatever she tried or who she saw, no one could help her.

This patient eventually became homebound because she couldn't function without becoming dizzy or falling down, and so she simply stopped leaving the relative safety of her home. She

94

was fearful of driving, being in cars, or going up and down stairs. She'd been my patient for some time but hadn't really mentioned any of this to me. I suddenly noticed that she began to look much older, and was much more withdrawn, constantly frowning and unhappy. I also started to notice that her mid-face area seemed to be collapsing somewhat. I later found out that she'd suffered from a number of other issues, including intense headaches and acid reflux.

This led me to do a complete TMD evaluation and through this I found even more signs and symptoms of TMD. She had a lot of dental work done over the years, and while it originally had looked very nice, it had begun to wear down over time and affect the way her teeth and smile looked. Once I did my workup and started a treatment plan to treat the TMD she'd clearly been suffering from, her vertigo symptoms soon disappeared. I was able to alleviate a lot of her symptoms and transform the way her face and smile looked. One of the most important results was that she started feeling comfortable with smiling again. The before and after pictures we took don't lie – she looks 20 years younger.

This patient's story is near and dear to my heart. It was an absolute success story and it reflects not only what I do, but why I do it. I want all of my patients to have a great looking smile, and I also want them to have the confidence and the comfort to smile. That, to me, is the definition of a truly beautiful smile.

ABOUT MICHAEL FIROUZIAN, DDS

Firouzian Dentistry
www.ColumbusCosmeticDental.com

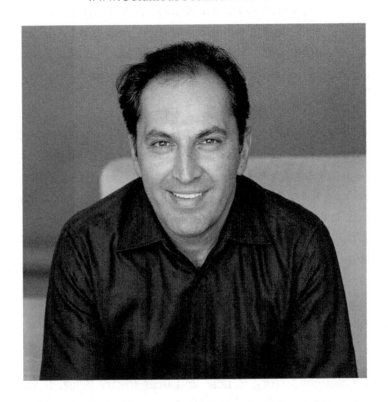

Dr. Michael "Mike" Firouzian receive a B.S. in Microbiology from the Ohio State University in 1987 and his D.D.S. in 1991. He also completed advanced training in general dentistry at the University of Florida College of Dentistry in 1992 and served as a clinical instructor as well as receiving a Master of Arts in Anthropology from The Ohio State University. Dr. Mike also has over 1,700 hours of continuing education, making him one of the nation's most highly trained cosmetic dentists.

Dr. Mike performs a wide range of dental procedures, including TMJ therapy, orthodontics and dental implants. He also works in the fields of reconstructive dentistry for those who have suffered trauma; sleep disorder diagnosis and treatment; and cosmetic procedures such as whitening, veneers and implants as well as therapeutic procedures such as bridges and crowns. His focus is on using dental techniques to solve a wide range of medical issues such as migraines and other related problems.

Dr. Mike holds fellowships with the Academy of General Dentistry and the International College of Craniomandibular Orthopedics as well as the Las Vegas Institute for Advanced Dental Studies. He is also a Top 3 Dentist in Columbus, Ohio and a contributor on Real Self.

As a general and family dentist, Dr. Mike has dedicated his life to providing patients with the exceptional dental care they need and deserve. He has extensive training in the areas of orthodontics, TMJ, obstructive sleep apnea and treatments of head and neck pain. He takes very seriously his responsibility to his patients, and is continually searching for answers to various medical problems, including those outside the field of dentistry.

There is no such thing as a "routine" visit with Dr. Mike! His entire clinical team works to evaluate and treat patients with physiologic and mercury-free dentistry, removing harmful amalgam fillings and replacing them with healthier, more natural materials. Dr. Mike and his team also work with advanced technique in addressing neuromuscular imbalances; bite and jaw alignment correction through restorative dentistry and orthodontics; Implant dentistry to replace one or more missing teeth that helps preserve integrity of the jaw bones and prevent bone loss that follows tooth loss; and management of obstructive sleep apnea (OSA) and its precursor, upper airway resistance syndrome (UARS) in both adults and children through various non-surgical techniques such as mandibular advancement devices (MADs), orthodontics, and restorative dentistry.

One special technique offered by Dr. Mike is Fountain of Youth® Dentures, a very special way to replace teeth and restore the person's youthful smile and facial features that can make them look ten or even twenty years younger. Dr. Mike also regularly collaborates with medical specialists such as cardiologists, pulmonologists, neurologists, allergists, ENT's, and others in comprehensively caring for patients.

Over the last two decades, he has considered many unanswered questions about patient problems and care, and these have driven his studies to seek answers he has not found readily available in the mainstream of dental practitioners. Dr. Mike has studied new procedures that provide better treatment options for his patients, and he has also encouraged that same level of training and understanding for his team.

STRAIGHT TALK ON ORTHODONTICS

E veryone wants a perfectly straight smile. Fortunately, the world of orthodontics offers a variety of options for patients of almost every age. Once considered a luxury where only the children of well-to-do families were seen with the metal grin, nowadays, orthodontic treatments are considered basic preventive care, are much more attainable with a myriad of options allowing for less treatment time as well as payment plays that accommodate a wide range of budget limitations. Additionally, a variety of modern colored braces are available to allow patients ways to express their individuality during the treatment. In today's society, there is very little standing in the way of achieving a beautiful and healthy smile and wellbeing that will last a lifetime.

The demographics of patients seeking orthodontic treatment have also been rapidly changing. In the past, most people sought orthodontic treatment for purely aesthetic reasons, either because they noticed portions of their smile were crooked or something didn't look quite right. Metals and bands were the norm and it was common for orthodontic treatments to take several years. Today, we have a renaissance of new technology with advanced diagnostic tools and treatment options that have significantly improved patient comfort, reduced treatment time and produced more holistic final outcomes. I have observed a shift where more and more adult patients are seeking orthodontic treatment and recognizing that along with aesthetic benefits, orthodontic treatment is crucial in improving the function of their teeth, oral health and ultimately, overall health and wellbeing.

ORTHODONTICS FOR FUNCTIONALITY AND HEALTH

Clearly, a lot of patients seek out orthodontic treatment to improve the look of their smile and boost their self-esteem. How often have we observed people shy away from public speaking or smiling due to misaligned teeth? Some people will not even publicly open their mouths because they are ashamed of their dental alignment. Orthodontic treatment will correct these problems and greatly enhance one's self esteem.

A great smile can light up one's face, make one appear younger and has many other desirable effects on one's appearance. In addition to all those cosmetic and psychological benefits, people may not be aware that a healthy and electrifying smile have other great health benefits in other areas of life as well. Smiling not only makes us more attractive, it releases endorphins, boosts our immune system, lowers our blood pressure, and changes our mood.

In addition, significant current research indicates that there are other dental health benefits that people can derive from treatment. Crooked or crowded teeth and imperfect bites allow for food and bacteria to become trapped and inaccessible to proper brushing and flossing. This contributes to plaque build-up, poor oral health, cavities, gum disease, which may later evolve into medical conditions that develop as an effect of the initial gum disease. The position of the teeth also has a dramatic impact on facial appearance and aging as well as on overall wellness through the influence the teeth and jaws have over tongue posture and the airway.

Individuals suffering from a bad bite, according to available studies and research today, can ultimately become victims of temporomandibular joint disorders (TMJD), which can cause a variety of symptoms including clicking, popping, ringing in the ears, and headaches.

More and more scientific evidence have demonstrated the intricate connection between their teeth, their oral health, and their overall health. Poorly-aligned teeth lead to poor bites and difficulty chewing, which can lead to poor digestion and gastrointestinal issues. It can also lead to teeth with excessive wear.

Studies have demonstrated that people with narrow maxillary arch are at increased risks of having constricted airways (since the upper jaw is closely connected to the nasal cavity) which may ultimately contribute to sleep apnea. These are just a few examples of how the state of a person's oral health can impact other areas of their health and their life.

Skilled orthodontists are well aware of problems that begin in the mouth that can later have devastating effects on the rest of the body. This is why the American Association of Orthodontists encourage parents to get their young children screened by an Orthodontist starting at 7 years old in order to prevent potential dental and skeletal problems and to plan ahead with treatment options. Proactive parents not only assist in their child's dental issues, but also contribute to the overall well-being of the child by preventing potential diseases occurring as the result of dental neglect. Orthodontics can help in these situations, giving individuals a solid bite and a beautiful smile at the same time.

NOTICING A CHANGE

A lot of patients are initially drawn to orthodontic treatment through recommendations made by their general dentists. However, as savvy consumers are getting more and more educated and more information are available to the public, more and more people are paying attention to their oral health and those noticing changes in their teeth or difficulties in their bite often prompt them to seek orthodontic treatment on their own.

Another key component of noticing dental changes is noticing speech difficulties. This is especially true for parents who notice their children have difficulty pronouncing certain words or phrases or experience some type of impediment to their speech. Most healthcare professionals understand that the position of teeth can drastically affect children and adolescents and how their speech develops. For example, individuals that have a large overbite, or teeth that are crowded or inclined, have difficulty getting their tongue in the correct position in between the teeth. We can easily tell a child have suffered these problems if they have an open bite, large overjet, overbite or from scalloping of their tongues caused by not having enough space for the tongue to rest in their correct position. We've found that a good deal of the speech problems that children – and adults – have stem from teeth and jaws that are improperly positioned in the mouth.

THE AESTHETIC 'BOOM'

Orthodontics is incredibly important in impacting the way people function in their daily lives by improving basic functions like chewing, speaking, as well as the health of their TMJ and airways. In recent decades, there has also been a boom when it comes to utilizing orthodontics to improve their total aesthetic outlook. More and more, people are aware of how their smile looks and how it shapes their social interactions, as well as how they feel about themselves. People have become more aware and concerned about the aesthetics of their smile.

The advent of Hollywood has brought about the 'Hollywood Smile' – and celebrities with beautiful pearly whites on television and in the public have played a big role in inspiring the general public to become more concerned about aesthetics. As people watch their favorite movies and television shows, they see these celebrities with beautiful smiles throughout all the media platforms, and they want to have the same "Hollywood smile". They want to be able to flaunt their smile and feel confident about how it looks to others, as well as to themselves.

Smiles are one of the simplest and, arguably, the most important way we initially connect with others. It is also a factor in how we maintain strong relationships with the people that are closest to us. A smile can say a lot about someone to others, especially to strangers or people that we meet for the first time. A smile is a first impression that tends to shape how we are viewed and perceived. Having a straight, white, beautiful smile is something that most people strive for. For this reason alone, a lot more people, especially adults, have been seeking orthodontic treatment to obtain a great smile.

THE BASICS OF BRACES

Braces are probably the most common form of treatment when people think of orthodontics for both aesthetic and functional reasons.

Braces are quite nifty of an invention. There are different components of braces that make them work. First, brackets are placed in the center of each tooth and each bracket has a specific prescription, based on the individual tooth and the needs of the patient. Then, there are archwires that are inserted through the brackets that apply continuous pressure to the teeth. This pressure causes the teeth to shift gradually over time into their ideal positions. This makes it easy for people with crooked teeth or those that have gaps between their teeth to get a healthier and more attractive smile by moving the teeth into a position where they align correctly.

Then, there are colorful little elastics, like mini rubber bands, that are placed on the braces to hold the archwires seated into the braces and keep everything together. These elastics are great because, much like your ability to choose the color of the wrapping on a cast, kids can choose different colored elastics to match their favorite outfits or even to make the braces less noticeable if they want.

Traditionally, an orthodontist will take a mold of a patient's teeth and then use that mold to make a cast. This cast is important because it helps the orthodontist carefully plan the treatment for each tooth and how it needs to be moved in order to get the teeth in the best possible position. After this, the position of each bracket can be determined to go along with the rest of the customized treatment. Some teeth may need to be tilted or moved in a very specific way, and this affects what bracket is used and how it is positioned on the tooth. Today, with the advent of digital smile design, the process starts with a 3D intraoral scan, which is much more comfortable for patients. With digital 3D models, the orthodontist can carefully design a smile that not only looks good, but has a functionally perfect bite using computer aided design. This is similar to an architect designing a beautiful skyscraper that is also structurally sound.

TYPES OF BRACES

There are a wide variety of braces that can be used. Even with traditional metal braces, there are possibly a hundred different brands. There are also more aesthetic options for adults or for individuals who are not enthusiastic about having metal braces that are more visible. The esthetic options include using clear ceramic brackets. These mimic metal braces in size and shape, but they are porcelain. They're basically crystalline, and are more difficult to see. This is a great option for any patient who wants something that is a little more aesthetic.

Another more innovative aesthetic option is the lingual braces, an option that we provide at my office in Torrance, CA. We are one of a few offices that offer this option. Lingual braces are applied behind the teeth, so you essentially get the best of both worlds: braces to correct your teeth that do not require much compliance and they are hidden so it's aesthetically pleasing. In my opinion, lingual braces function more efficiently than traditional braces because every aspect of the design is done by an orthodontist using computer-aided design, the bracket placements are accomplished using 3D printed jigs, and wires precisely bent by robots. They are more challenging for orthodontists to put on because it's obviously more difficult to work on the inside of a patient's teeth. However, they are just as effective as traditional braces, if not more so, while being completely invisible to the outside.

TREATMENT PLANS FOR BRACES

Every patient has a customized treatment plan for their braces. Generally, the orthodontist will see each patient every four weeks to check their progress and to see if any adjustments need to be made. There are some orthodontists that can apply advanced techniques which allow patients to come in only every eight to twelve weeks. For example, there are self-ligating brackets used with body heat-activated nickel-titanium memory wire that can be used to make the need for adjustment appointments less often. These memory wire are programmed with the patient's ideal arch form, and using the patient's body heath slowly return to their pre-programmed shape, gently moving their teeth into their correct position.

At my practice, we utilize digital smile design which involves a 3D intraoral scan which creates a 3D model of a patient's teeth. This replaces the traditional mold that most orthodontists use and allows us to digitally design the model and properly treatment plan the patient's mouth. Using digital tools, we can better plan the treatment using virtual guides, automatic measurement tools, and virtually fitting brackets on the teeth in virtual space and formulate different treatment plans before selecting the best plan custom-tailored to the individual patient. We can also 3D print jigs that can be used to precisely place brackets to their perfect position, and use robot bent memory wire that is customized to the patient's treatment plan, which decreases the need for more frequent patient visits, while speeding up treatment.

The amount of time braces need to be worn depends on each patient and their specific needs. A few years ago, the average amount of time braces are worn is typically 24-30 months, or around two or two and a half years. Today, an orthodontist using the more advanced techniques available now can cut the time down significantly to between 12 and 18 months.

ADVANCED TECHNIQUES

It's important to note that the use of the advanced techniques I mentioned above – as well as a host of other new techniques –

requires additional training on the orthodontist's part. All dentists go through extensive training, but orthodontists go through additional training (and an additional residency) to better understand the jaw and how it works. It usually takes about two to three years of additional orthodontic specialty training on top of general dental education. As a graduate, the orthodontist then becomes board eligible. In addition, currently, only about 25% of orthodontists are board certified by the American Board of Orthodontics (ABO). The ABO certification process signifies a unique achievement—a significant step beyond the two to three years of advanced education required for a dentist to become a specialist in orthodontics. The process requires the orthodontist to demonstrate actual accomplishments in patient care with detailed case reports on the treatment provided for a broad range of patient problems. Board certification is a voluntary achievement that not all orthodontists choose to pursue. In order to become board certified by the ABO, an individual orthodontist has his/her patient cases thoroughly examined using strict criteria and undergoes an extensive interview process by a highly-respected panel of examiners to demonstrate their orthodontic knowledge, clinical skills and judgment. This requires the orthodontist to stay up to date with the latest cutting-edge advanced techniques. I'm proud to be included in the select group of board-certified orthodontists who are not only looking to straighten teeth, but we also measure the functionality of the teeth, how they come together, and what position they need to be in to not only look good but also to help the patient's mouth function properly. There are dozens of measurements we use to make sure this happens, many of which greatly aided by 3D smile design. And the advanced techniques we employ allow us to find the most efficient way to achieve a beautiful, functional smile for our patients.

More revolutionary orthodontists can use advanced techniques equipment such as a 3D cone beam CT scan to better visualize the patient's teeth in 3D and diagnose more complex issues, and 3D intraoral scans to build 3D models of the patient's teeth and also to aid in diagnosing the issues and creating the best treatment plan for the patient. Using this advanced technique, we are able to anticipate how the teeth will look at the end of treatment before we even begin the process of designing and applying the braces. It allows us to effectively and efficiently customize each patient's treatment, which saves a lot of time, as well as cutting down on the number of visits necessary for a patient to complete treatment.

In my practice, we have all of the 3D technology in our office, including a 3D intraoral scanner, 3D printer, 3D cone beam CT (3D x-rays), and sophisticated computer aided smile design software. All of this technology enables us to provide our patients the very best treatment plans, to execute specific and customized treatment they need to improve final results, improve safety, and to cut down both the frequency of visits and the length of time patients need to wear their braces.

We use a lot of different therapies to accelerate a patient's treatment. There is the OrthoPulse which utilizes the photobiomodulation phenomenon to achieve light-accelerated orthodontics. These light in the near infrared spectrum have been shown to promote cell metabolism and allow the body to regenerate, heal, and reduce inflammation and pain. The device uses low levels of light energy to stimulate the bone surrounding the roots of teeth to remodel and facilitate tooth movement.

Another option that we have available is periodontally accelerated osteogenic orthodontics (PAOO). A common brand is Propel, which involves micro-osteoperforation. Basically, the procedures will create micro-perforations in the bone, which increases bone turnover and accelerates teeth movement. It's incredibly useful, specifically for adults who are generally more difficult to treat because their bones are much denser than those of children.

Furthermore, another option currently on the market is the AcceleDent which mobilizes the teeth, making them shift into place more quickly using vibration.

Generally, acceleration devices act by stimulating the bone remodeling process that involves increasing bone cell turnover activities to increase the movement of patients' teeth. This requires activating the osteoclast (a bone cell that resorbs bone tissue during growth and healing) and osteoblast (a cell that secretes matrix proteins that help form bone tissue) activities. Engaging in this therapy allows us expedite treatment times for our patients.

ARE BRACES PAINFUL?

This is a very common question in the mind of our patients. Braces, in and of themselves, do not cause pain, but the stiff archwires that are placed into the braces may cause pressure as the teeth are being moved. With modern braces, we can use soft body heat activated memory wires that apply a gentler, but continuous force. These are a big improvement over traditional steel wires where the patients may experience higher initial pain during the initial adjustment when the orthodontist bent the wire every 2-4 weeks during regular adjustment. With memory wire, the patient will likely experience very minimal discomfort over the first two-weeks adjustment period. After that, the memory wire will apply the same gentle constant force throughout the remaining 90% of the treatment. In some cases, metal bands on the four teeth in the very back of the mouth – 2 upper and 2 lower

–are used as anchors for the braces. Sometimes, putting the bands on can cause some discomfort because they are snug and fitted all the way down to the gum. However, separators are generally used before the fitting of the bands to lessen the discomfort. The rest of the process of application isn't painful. Most of the discomfort is associated with two aspects of braces: the borders of the brackets and the movement that the braces cause. With traditional braces that are metal, they can rub against the inside of the patient's mouth and cause irritation and pain. However, once the skin inside the mouth adjusts to the brackets being there, a lot of the discomfort subsides.

The movement of the teeth is oftentimes compared to a baby teething. When babies start to get teeth, they feel the movement and pressure of the teeth trying to break through the bone and gums. With braces, the teeth are, of course, constantly moving. However, they are moving at a fairly slow pace, so it's not drastic nor do all the movements happen at once. We have different options available to reduce any discomfort that the patient may experience.

KEEPING BRACES CLEAN

Keeping braces clean is a little more intricate than just brushing your teeth. That, of course, is still the first thing that should be done. However, there have been a lot of inventions designed specifically to help patients with braces to keep them clean. Ultrasonic vibrating toothbrushes such as Sonicare can be a great tool to really get in-between the teeth and around the braces. There are also specific orthodontic kits that include small interproximal brushes that allow patients to clean under the wire and around the brackets. There are also floss threaders that make it easier to get floss under the arch wires making it easier to floss.

ELIGIBILITY FOR BRACES

Most people are good candidates for braces and there are very few people who are not good candidates. People who have poor oral health or serious decay are about the only people that shouldn't get braces or should get these issues treated before pursuing braces. If their oral health is suffering to a great enough degree, gum problems might also be something that needs to be treated. In that case, of course, we'd refer them to a periodontist to get the issue resolved. We like to keep an open line of communication with the patient's primary care dentist or periodontist to make sure that they're cleared to get orthodontic treatment.

THE COST OF BRACES

Most PPO dental insurances offer a lifetime maximum for orthodontic treatment. They typically cover orthodontic treatments, which includes braces. The actual cost of braces varies by region, by state, and from one doctor to another. It's also going to depend on the specific needs of each patient. However, if I were to give conservative estimates, I'd say that phase one of treatment, which is early interceptive care before applying braces, ranges about $2000-3,900. For phase two of care, which involves the braces and teeth alignment and making sure the bite is correct, ranges between $5,500 to $6,500 in total.

HOW BRACES MAKE A DIFFERENCE - THE STORY OF JOHNNY

I'd like to share a story about a patient who got braces that illustrates how braces can totally transform a person's life.

Johnny is a patient that I will never be able to forget. When I first met him during his orthodontic consult, he was about 10 years old. I knew that there was something a little bit different about him. He was very bright, but, he was also incredibly reserved. There was a kind of heaviness about him, like something was weighing him down. His mother told me that he'd been begging her for braces since he was about 6. The primary issue had been his family's financial situation – they just didn't have the resources to get him braces. He was very mature for his age. I could tell that something was bothering him from the moment I met him.

It wasn't until later on, during other visits, as I got to know him personally that he opened up to me, He told me that from a young age he'd been bullied at school because his front teeth stuck out awkwardly. He was teased constantly and ruthlessly. I also learned that he'd never told his parents about the bullying or the extent with which it had been done. He held it in and that, I realized, was the heaviness about him that I'd sensed during that first visit.

He finally got braces after begging his parents incessantly. His expression on the day that his braces came off that will always stay with me. When he first looked in the mirror and saw his new smile, it was like a cloud that had surrounded him was lifted. He was beaming, smiling from ear to ear. It was the happiest he'd ever been. He laughed and he cried. Every visit after that – I saw him for about a year or two after the braces – I saw his confidence growing and his outlook became brighter.

His mother noticed, too. She told me that she saw him being happier, more outgoing and became involved with his peers and school activities. His grades even improved. His mother had told me that when they first came in, though he was incredibly smart, he was getting C's and D's. As his confidence grew and the bullying stopped, he was able to focus, his opinion of himself changed, and he became a straight-A student. He ended up joining the football team in high school, he developed a great friend group, and when he graduated, he ended up going on to an Ivy-League school.

The beautiful thing about Johnny's case is that I was able to observe his total transformation from a troubled boy to a happy, confident young man. The reality is that although his teeth did need work, it was truly all about how he looked and how that affected his perception of himself, as well as how others perceived and treated him. The change to his smile helped him shift his perception – and the perception of others - from negative to positive. It was a total personality change. It might be one of the most important and significant cases I've ever had the privilege to treat.

Johnny's case helped me in another way – it changed the way I interacted with 'my kids' (I treat all of my young patients like my 'kids'). I began to make a pointed effort to treat all kids with the utmost respect. I also started screening these patients for a history of bullying. It's important that we never underestimate how a child's smile impacts their life, their growth, their potential and ability to reach it fully. This has been a really great transformation for me and my team, making sure that every kid we treat gets the best orthodontic treatment, but also the best total care that we can possibly give.

THE BASICS ABOUT CLEAR ALIGNERS

Clear aligners are a great alternative to traditional braces. Clear aligners are essentially an appliance that is removable. It snaps onto the teeth and is designed to help the teeth move. These are really great for patients who want a straight smile without the metal and wires in their mouth. These aligners are designed for people who are socially active and want to be discreet about their orthodontic treatment. I see a lot of patients who are getting married soon or preparing for other important events. Aligners make it possible for them to remove the appliance before the event or for pictures.

Aligners function similarly to traditional braces in that they move a person's teeth. However, the execution is different. Aligners, as I mentioned, are appliances, a series of clear trays that snap on and fit snugly to the teeth. They are made from traditional dental molds or with 3D intraoral scans like those we use in my practice. The great thing about using the 3D technology is that we can digitally create a model of the patient's teeth and then create the aligners around the model. We incorporate the specific prescription to each tray, just as we do with the brackets and their placement when using traditional braces.

Aligners are growing in popularity and a lot of people are probably familiar with some of the brands that are used, such as Invisalign® and ClearCorrect®. We also use our 3D printing technology to make our very own customized clear aligners. Invisalign® has been around the longest; it's very popular, and provide great treatment planning tools to the orthodontists. ClearCorrect® came onto the market a little later, but offer an affordable alternative.

TREATMENT PLAN FOR ALIGNERS

Aligners work by slowly moving crooked teeth a little bit with each set of aligners. They are designed with pressure points that push the teeth closer to their ideal position. The treatment plan at Breeze Orthodontics starts with 3D scan to create a 3D model of the patient's teeth, jaw, and gums. We segment them into 3D objects, which we can manipulate using 3D smile design software.

I create a 3D animation to establish what their specific treatment plan needs to look like, determining what each tray needs to look like, frame by frame. I pay very close attention to the limits of the teeth and the patient's mouth, including how they're situated in the jawbone, in order to avoid any damage. Once the treatment plan is created and approved, it's sent to the lab for manufacturing.

The frequency of patient visits depends a lot on the patient and their individual needs. In general, we're able to see these patients a lot less frequently. Usually, we have them come in every 12 weeks or so. We're able to do this because the entire treatment plan and all of its stages are planned ahead of time. We can even show patients what their teeth are expected to look like at every step along the way and what we expect them to look like when the process is finished. That's one of the greatest advantages of using the 3D technology, as well as using clear aligners, which allow the patient to see what their teeth look like and how they are changing. For most patients, the treatment plan is completed in six to 18 months. It's important to mention that aligners need to be worn about 22 hours a day to ensure consistent pressure on the teeth so that they move the way the treatment plan designed them to.

The primary advantages of clear aligners are that they are less visible, they can be removed, and they really help cut down the length of time that orthodontics are necessary. They're also less restrictive on a person's diet because the patients don't wear them when they eat. They also have the upper hand when it comes to less pain, because they don't involve metal or wires in the mouth.

GOOD CANDIDATES FOR ALIGNERS

As with braces, pretty much all patients are good candidates for aligners. There are only a few caveats. First, as with traditional braces, if a person has gum disease or decay, these issues need to be addressed before they could be considered for aligners. Also, if patients need structural or skeletal treatment, that should be addressed first. These are challenging to do with aligners because of the moving target the shifting jaw lines and growing teeth presents. However, with all of the advances in technology, we're actually able to incorporate some of the skeletal treatment in with the aligners.

However, if there are individuals suffering from jaw asymmetry, they may need temporary anchorage devices (TADs). These are basically bone stabilizers used to correct asymmetry. Also, patients with a severe overbite or underbite will need another adjunct like a skeletal corrector. These individuals need more treatment than just aligners.

The final caveat deals with responsibility. It's imperative that a patient is responsible and is willing to follow the rules around when to keep the aligners in and when to take them out.

THE COST OF ALIGNERS

Most PPO dental insurances offer benefits that cover orthodontic treatments like aligners. Putting an average dollar amount on the cost of aligners, I'd say that you're looking at a general range of about $4,500 to $7,000. There are some areas of the country where the cost might go as high as $10,000.

Something to note: some places will charge significantly less because not all orthodontic offices offer name brand aligners. We personally like Invisalign® because of their 20-year history and their 3D software offers one of the best customizability of the treatment. Other brands have recently emerged offering cheaper and possibly less reliable alternatives.

ALIGNERS IN ACTION

I'd like to share another patient story, this one showing how transformative aligners can be.

May came to see me. She had a gap in between her teeth. She'd had braces before. She said, "I'm an adult. I don't want braces again". The gap was really bothering her. She let me know that she was having a lot of trouble with eating - food was getting stuck in the gap. She was also at the age where she was looking for someone that she could spend the rest of her life with. We decided that aligners would be the very best option for her.

When we did her consult, I told her that the treatment could last for about 12 to 18 months. When she came in to get the scan done, she told me that she'd found someone, gotten engaged, and that she was going to be getting married in eight months. I was able to customize her treatment using a very efficient plan that closed her gap nicely. The bonus was that her Invisalign® treatment ended right before her wedding. She was beautiful on her wedding day, and she had a beautiful smile to go with it. She was able to smile with confidence. She truly glowed. It was such a wonderful transformation to witness.

THE IMPORTANCE OF ORTHODONTIC TREATMENT

Orthodontics can have a major impact on a person's smile. While it's incredibly important to correct skeletal issues, gum disease, and decay, orthodontics get teeth into the right position, which is structurally important, but also cosmetically important. I've said it before but it bears repeating: having a straight smile plays a huge role in how people perceive themselves, how they feel about themselves, and how successfully they interact with others. All of these things affect a person's self-esteem, how they function at school or work, and their ability to reach their full potential. It's about giving patients a smile they are proud of, boosting their level of confidence.

I feel it's also important to reiterate that it's so vital to pay special attention to children who need orthodontic treatment. Children and adolescents are at the point in their lives where they are developing their identity, making connections with friends, constructing who they are. Orthodontic treatment does more than reposition their teeth. It gives them a great smile. It helps to build their confidence and lays a foundation of positivity when it comes to how they feel about themselves. This is crucial if they are going to make choices in their lives that are positive.

ONE FINAL STORY

I'd like to share one final story that, like the others, shows what a really significant difference orthodontic treatment can make in a person's life.

Heidi is one of my older patients. She was 55 when she first came to see me. She was kind of similar to Johnny. She had a heaviness about her that I noticed right away. She told me that she always avoided smiling. She said that smiling was something she'd wanted to be able to do for a long time, ever since she was a child. Her teeth had always been very crooked, but because of her family's financial situation, she wasn't able to get braces as a child. She worked hard as an adult, taking on three jobs just to be able to get braces. Being able to smile was so important to her, and the fact that she hated her crooked teeth so much impacted how she functioned at school, at work, and in social situations.

When she'd finally saved up enough money, she came in for a consult. We worked with her and were able to offer her financing to help cover the costs of treatment.

Once Heidi's treatment was finished, her entire personality was transformed. She was 56 when her treatment ended, but she acted almost like she was 16 again. Her demeanor changed. She immediately got a new hairdo and started putting on makeup. We were able to see this transformation take place throughout her treatment, and how her whole life seemed to change once we were done. It was almost as if her life hadn't really started until we were done with her treatment. Heidi didn't get just a great smile. She got a brand-new life and a new outlook to go with it.

Heidi's story illustrates really well how orthodontic treatment can totally change a person's life. Her story is a great example of why I do what I do. I'm happy to give patients a more functional bite, of course. But the true blessing is being able to give them a beautiful smile and to see how it completely changes their lives in a positive way.

ABOUT RITA Y. CHUANG, DDS

Breeze Orthodontics
www.BreezeOrtho.com

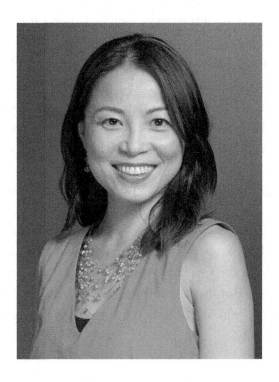

Dr. Rita Chuang is an American Board of Orthodontics Certified Orthodontist who is passionate about improving smiles and empowering patients to live life to the fullest. Her background includes degrees from Cornell University and the University of Pennsylvania, where she served as Clinical Director. She also attended the University of Southern California and holds degrees in dentistry and Specialty certification in Orthodontics. She focuses her professional efforts on cutting-edge orthodontic treatments to provide patients with life-changing smile and healthy improvements in bite, airways and temporomandibular joints.

Dr. Chuang offers patients the latest in cutting-edge orthodontic techniques, including lingual braces and Invisalign® as well as cosmetic and preventative treatments that enhance smiles and create confidence. Along with her efficient staff, she helps patients obtain the smiles they deserve through new dental advances and utilizes the newest and best treatments available to ensure that all patients are able to obtain the smile they want and deserve.

Dr. Chuang offers both children and adults treatment for a variety of orthodontic problems, including overlapping teeth; rotated teeth; spaces between teeth; protruding teeth or overbite, and problems with misalignment. She also offers preventative care and treatment for many types of oral and dental issues like TMJ, sleep apnea, and snoring problems. Dr. Chuang and her highly capable team ensure that every patient is given personalized care that meets his or her individual needs and provides appropriate treatment options for all types of orthodontic issues.

Dr. Chuang spends hundreds of hours each year studying the latest in dental and orthodontic procedures. She also serves on numerous national orthodontic boards, dental societies and philanthropic organizations. Dr. Chuang and her staff are dedicated to providing professional, competent and compassionate care to all patients.

CONSEQUENCES OF MISSING TEETH

In the United States alone, there are nearly 200 million people missing at least one tooth, and more than 30 million people who have lost all their teeth. That's a staggering statistic. This is a growing problem just due to the fact that people are living longer, and that people are more prone to losing teeth as they age. There are a number of reasons for that, for example the side effects of taking certain medications that can have a negative effect on your oral health.

The issue of missing teeth is not just a cosmetic issue. It's much more than that. The consequences of missing teeth adversely affect not only your oral health but your overall health, both physical and emotional. Often, people are unaware of just how far-reaching the consequences of missing teeth can be.

I had a woman in her mid-50s come to see me. She had been in a workplace accident and had a number of her teeth knocked out. She was so dramatically impacted by this accident, and the effect that it had on her smile, that she did not want people to see her. She stopped socializing, and eventually, it got to the point where she would hardly ever leave her house. She stopped working entirely and had lost a lot of weight because of her inability to chew and was in poor overall health – both mentally and physically.

She ended up finding me and my team, and I knew as soon as I talked with her and examined her that implants would be a great option. The major issue was the fact that it took years for her workman's compensation claim to be approved. Once the approval finally came through, I was able to offer her an instant change. She was the perfect candidate for the All-on-4® implant procedure. A procedure where we are able to give her teeth in one visit!

The day the implants were placed, we attached the new teeth to the implants, and it immediately changed the look of her smile and her face. Within just a few short hours, we were able to completely solve the issues that had been plaguing her for years. When she picked up the mirror and saw her brand-new smile, she cried. She was so full of happiness and joy. It was a total and totally beautiful transformation. And it really turned her whole life around. She began going out socially again and really enjoying living a full life. Getting her smile fixed changed her world.

THE CAUSES OF MISSING TEETH

The consequences of missing teeth can be very far-reaching. Missing teeth eventually cause your facial muscles to deteriorate, changing your facial appearance. Obviously, missing teeth affect your ability to chew food. As you lose the ability to chew your food properly, that in turn affects your ability to digest food and absorb the nutrients from food that your body needs. Many people aren't aware of the fact that the digestive process starts in your mouth. If you can't chew your food properly, then your stomach can't break the food down properly because the digestive process didn't start properly.

There are two primary causes of tooth loss. The first is the terminal effects of periodontal disease. Periodontal disease, by definition, is a bacterial infection that occurs under the gum, usually as a result of improper care and cleaning, but that can also be triggered by various medications and medical conditions, which diabetes is a major factor. Periodontal disease is somewhat like an invasion of your oral system that gradually causes it to break down.

To understand periodontal disease more easily, think about the human body as a closed system that wants to remain closed. For example, if you get a cut on your finger, then your body's system becomes open. To fix this, your body will attempt to heal the cut and close the system again. This is the major way that the body stops infections and the spreading of a disease. The mouth of the human body is also a closed system, with your gums attached to your teeth so that there's a seal there. Nothing can get into or out of the gum without force or damage to the gum, the tooth, or both.

Once you get periodontal disease, that seal is broken making it easier for other debris and bacteria to infiltrate and cause infections and inflammation. This causes breakdown of the gum attachments around the tooth and eventually bone loss around the tooth and in the jaw. When enough bone loss occurs, the teeth become so loose they fall out. Basically, your body, in an attempt to close the wound and close the system again, wants to extract the tooth naturally. Just like a splinter you get in your finger which becomes infected the body wants the splinter out and once the splinter is removed the infection is gone and the wound is healed. Once the tooth is gone, the gum does close over it and now the wound is closed.

The second major cause of tooth loss is decay. Decay can happen for a variety of reasons, but the primary reason is nutrition and lack of proper care of the teeth. We should strive to prevent decay or to catch it early before major damage is done and correct it once it happens. Cavities, caused by decaying of the teeth, require fillings or root canals to prevent the decay from spreading further. Without this corrective treatment, the tooth will continue to decay and will eventually get to a point where it can no longer be fixed and will need to be extracted to prevent infection in the gums or in the jaw bones. There is a reason why you are recommended to see your dentist at least twice a year. It's all based on prevention and catching problems when they are small.

I can't stress enough the importance of regular dental visits. Some people won't go to a dentist unless they're having significant pain, but the problem is that by the time you experience pain, there's usually already been substantial damage. However, if you see your dentist regularly, they can evaluate and repair problems long before it reaches that point.

Other causes of missing teeth include trauma, such as a car accident or fall. Often diseases that aren't directly related to tooth decay and side effects of certain medications can cause it or tooth loss. Many elderly people are taking chronic medication for conditions like high cholesterol, heart disease, or high blood pressure. There are also people who are under chemotherapy or radiation for cancer. These medications and treatments all have side effects, and the major one is dry mouth. When you have dry mouth, that changes the pH of your saliva, and the oral environment becomes less resistant to the bacteria that cause decay.

You could have great teeth your whole life, and once you reach your 60s or 70s, after being on medication for a while, you notice lots of decay in your mouth. If that decay isn't fixed at an early stage, then there is a good chance that you're going to end up losing teeth. This is an increasing cause of tooth loss simply because people, in general, are taking a lot more medication these days.

ONE CASE OF MISSING TEETH

Before I continue, I'd like to share the story of a patient I treated. It's a good reflection of how missing teeth affect a person's aesthetics, and how that affects other areas of their lives.

I had a patient come to see me, a very personable lady in her mid-70s. Her lower teeth were in poor shape and several were missing. She worked as a waitress, a profession that generally requires a good deal of interaction with others. When she showed up at my office, one of the first things that she mentioned was the fact that she was very self-conscious about her smile and that her customers often asked her why she wasn't really talking to them or smiling. The simple fact was that she hated the way her smile looked and was scared to even open her mouth, despite the fact that she's a very sociable lady.

In one visit, I was able to correct and replace her lower teeth. It was a genuinely remarkable transformation. When she came back for her follow-up appointment, she gave me and my staff hugs and kisses, and her smile beamed. "You have no idea how this has impacted my life," she said. "I'm so happy, so outgoing now. Do you know what the best part is? My customers have noticed and I'm getting much larger tips now!"

This woman's new smile gave her back the ability to be sociable, friendly, and also had a dramatic impact on her work life.

BRUCE SEIDNER, DDS

The Aesthetics and Impact of Missing Teeth

It's fairly obvious, as the above story illustrates, that missing teeth pose aesthetic issues, but also affect more than just the smile itself. When you lose teeth and consequently lose supporting bone around the teeth, you lose portions of your facial structure. To provide a really clear example, consider an extreme case where a person has lost all of their teeth. The chin begins to move closer to the nose and the face takes on a noticeably sunken-in appearance. In less extreme cases, where you lose teeth individually, or a few here and there, the jaw muscles and the jaw bone begin to sag around the spaces where the teeth no longer are. This is why it's so important to address missing teeth as soon as possible, to prevent bone loss.

It's important to understand that fixing missing teeth and restoring a person's smile is about so much more than simply appearance. The way a person's smile looks affects how they interact with others, how they feel about themselves, and this affects how they take care of themselves in general. People with missing teeth hide their smile or don't smile at all. I've had many patients tell me things like, "It's been years since I've been able to smile. I don't want to smile. I'm embarrassed. I have no self-confidence. Sometimes I feel hopeless. The pain that I get sometimes from not having the teeth takes away from my quality of life."

Some people start to feel hopeless, like there's no solution for the way they feel, and become severely depressed. A great smile boosts self-confidence and is a key part of a person's self-image. This is the real reason that, aesthetically, it's so vital to correct a smile that's been negatively affected by missing or damaged teeth.

128

SHIFTING BITE

There are structural issues that arise from missing teeth, namely, a shifting bite. In the natural design of the jaw, our upper and lower teeth are all created to fit together in a perfect, functional system. When you begin to lose teeth, that system is altered and teeth begin to shift. They can start to lean in or out, rotate, or other teeth around the missing teeth will move because the missing teeth are not there to provide stability and keep everything in its proper place. The upper teeth will drop down or the lower teeth will shift upward. And all of those changes that missing teeth cause eventually themselves cause more bone loss and more teeth to be lost.

Even small changes in the alignment of your bite can lead to other problems, including issues with the jaw joints that can cause headaches, clicking, jaw pain, and basically, your bite just doesn't feel right. Once the bite shifts, the muscles that control the bite shift as well, and they try to compensate for each other. The resulting negative effects on your jaw muscles and joints can be very far-reaching, including not just jaw aches but neck aches and shoulder aches as well. That's because everything becomes misaligned after a while.

Clearly, as your bite shifts, it becomes more difficult to properly chew your food, especially when your chewing teeth in the back are missing. You can't chew and crush your food effectively, and I've even had patients come to me with painful lacerations on their gums because their gums are taking the brunt of the impact from the chewing action. In addition the pressure that the underlying bone takes causes further bone loss. As I mentioned earlier, the inability to adequately chew your food then becomes an issue in terms of nutrition.

The first step in digestion is proper chewing, where the food remains in the mouth long enough to be broken up with the teeth and then broken down by saliva before it is swallowed and enters the stomach. The more whole that the food is when it enters your stomach, then the harder it is for the stomach to break down. This is harsh on the stomach itself and takes a toll on your entire system because it means you don't get all the nutrients out of the food you've eaten.

SOLUTIONS FOR MISSING TEETH

There are a number of options to solve the problem of missing teeth. Of course, there are some people who choose not to do anything. This is always an option, however, because of the serious visual and physical problems I've mentioned above, it's not an option that I'd ever recommend.

If you have two good teeth on either side of a missing tooth, a bridge is a potential option. Basically, the good teeth are prepared and used as anchors, and a row of crowns is put in – one to fill in the gap, and two on the two adjacent good teeth. The disadvantage with this option is that it requires the filing down and damaging of perfectly good teeth in order to repair the gap made by the missing tooth. And because the root of that missing tooth is still missing in the jaw bone, bone loss can still occur in the jaw around the area of the missing tooth.

Dentures – either full or partial – are another option. That restores your bite for a certain period of time, however, over time as the denture is worn, the bone support underneath begins to wear away. Eventually, patients that use dentures for an extended period of time end up with even more bone loss.

Dentures are, essentially, plastic trays with teeth that sit over your gums and act in place of your teeth. The major problem with dentures, aside from their inability to prevent bone loss, is the fact that they are prone to shift and move with or without out adhesive. With upper dentures that cover the whole roof of your mouth, you lose your sense of taste. Some people can't even wear upper dentures because they cause some people to gag since the denture plate goes so far back on the palate.

The one advantage that an upper denture has over a lower denture is that you have more surface area to help it stay in place. Most people have to use the paste and glue to help anchor it securely. The lower denture, because of the limited surface area, are hard to keep from moving, even with adhesive.

Problems can occur when replacing missing teeth with removable devices such as, it's not comfortable and it doesn't address the issue of bone loss in the jaw. Also, it wears on the teeth around the removable appliance, so that they eventually decay and they become compromised.

The best option we've found for missing teeth, the best and most effective treatment technology, is to place dental implants.

A dental implant is a titanium screw that mimics, or basically takes the place of, the root of a tooth. Getting implants is a surgical procedure where the implant is placed into your jawbone and allowed to heal, and becomes part of the jawbone. Once it's healed, a post called an implant abutment goes on top of it. That sticks out through your gum into your mouth. On top of the abutment, we put a crown, which gives you the appearance of a natural tooth. That's an implant in its simplest form. It is critical to address missing teeth as soon as possible. Once a lot of bone has been lost, implants may no longer be a viable treatment option.

Implant technology has improved rapidly over the years and has a very high success rate. One of the major advances in implant technology is the "All-on-4"[®] procedure, where four implants are placed to hold restorations for an entire set of upper or lower teeth. For individuals who've already experienced bone loss, the All-on-4[®] system is a good implant option because we find and place the implants in areas where there is enough bone to sustain them. This is a revolutionary procedure for people who's teeth are failing and do not want to wear a denture. It gives you a new smile and the ability to eat again in one day!

So, implants can be used to fix a single missing tooth, a few teeth, or even all of a person's teeth. Once the implant has integrated with the bone, an artificial tooth – usually a crown - is affixed to the top of the implant. This allows the height of the bone to be maintained – the bone doesn't shrink – and restores the bite to what it should be. Ultimately, implants are the best option in terms of preventing bone loss and restoring the bite and smile to what it needs to be and to what patients would like it to be.

IMPLANTS IN ACTION

To better illustrate just how life-changing and successful implants can be, I'd like to share one more story, this one about a very recent patient of mine.

I had a case just this morning, a young man who, as the result of living a hard life and not getting proper, regular dental care, had significant problems of tooth decay and tooth loss even though he was only in his 30's Overall, he was a very attractive man, except for his smile. But the appearance of his smile was so bad that it was affecting the whole quality of his life.

Like most people with missing teeth, he was embarrassed, felt self-conscious, and had low self-esteem. Because of his missing teeth, his bite had shifted and had developed what we call an under-bite, where his lower teeth came in front of his upper teeth sought of the way a bulldog bite. In addition to negatively affecting his appearance, it also caused major functional problems in chewing his food.

This morning, we removed all of his broken and decayed teeth and we placed five implants in his upper arch. We gave him a brand-new smile that functions better than his old teeth did. His mother actually cried and hugged us all. She thanked us all for giving her son his life back. He was absolutely amazed, and said, "This is incredible. I can't believe you guys did this."

I think that story illustrates the severe negative consequences of missing teeth, but more importantly it also shows how dentists are able to fix the problem of missing teeth with treatment procedures such as dental implants. The opportunity to address these issues, to help restore my patients' ability to function and enjoy life to the fullest is exactly why I do what I do. It's about so much more than changing smiles. It's about changing lives.

ABOUT BRUCE SEIDNER, DDS

Seidner Dentistry
www.RandolphNJDentist.com

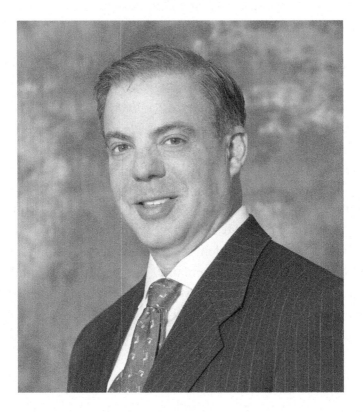

As a child, Dr. Seidner was always fearful of going to the dentist. It was his quest to find a better way for others to feel more comfortable and at ease in the dental chair. It was this desire to help others that led him to choose dentistry as a profession.

Dr. Bruce Seidner knew he could offer a better way to treat patients without fear. He founded his dental practice committed to "cater to cowards," training his entire team to offer a gentle dental experience. The mission of Dr. Seidner and his team is to go above and beyond to make his patients feel comfortable and relaxed as well as to strive to provide virtually painless dentistry.

Dr. Seidner is a 1984 graduate of Emory Dental School in Atlanta, Georgia. He earned his fellowship in The Academy of General Dentistry in 2001. He has also participated in extensive postgraduate courses in orthodontics as well as sedation and implant dentistry. He has trained with some of the country's most prominent sedation dental specialists and is a member of the Dental Organization for Conscious Sedation. By offering conscious sedation dentistry, Dr. Seidner can give hope to highly anxious patients whose fear prevents them from receiving necessary dental treatment.

Dr. Seidner has always had attention to detail and desire to be the best. When he learned of the revolutionary procedure All on 4®, which offers an entire arch of teeth corrected in one day, he set out to become one of the leading clinicians of this procedure in the country. This concept provides a fixed bridge for patients who are about to lose all their teeth or have dentures. He passionately feels dentures are a thing of the past and no one needs to suffer from missing teeth. By offering his patients "teeth in one day," he can significantly improve their smile, health, self-esteem, and quality of life.

Seidner Dentistry was one of the first offices in New Jersey to sponsor Dentistry from the Heart, a national non-profit organization dedicated to providing free dental care to those who need it. In the years that Dr. Seidner has hosted this event, he and his staff have helped over 1,500 people with free dental care. In addition to various charitable drives the office organizes, his favorite event is the annual Halloween Candy Buyback. Halloween candy is purchased from the community and packaged and sent to the troops overseas. The overwhelming appreciation from our troops is extremely rewarding. He was selected as Chabad's Man of the Year in 2013, an honor bestowed on outstanding members in the community.

FILLING THE GAPS WITH DENTAL IMPLANTS

D ental implants employ state of the art technology to offer patients truly remarkable improvements in their appearance, how well their teeth function, and in how they feel about themselves. Replacing missing teeth using dental implants can do more than just give you back a beautiful smile – they can also make a big difference in your self-esteem, self-confidence, and your overall happiness in life.

I'd like to share a story with you about one of my patients, one that I think does a good job of helping people understand the difference dental implant dentistry can make.

This patient was a young kid who happened to dance with the wrong girl one night at a nightclub. The girl's boyfriend and some of his friends took the kid outside and beat him up very severely, finishing things off by kicking his face into the curb of the sidewalk. He was in the hospital for about a month. They had knocked out most of his teeth. The poor kid told his grandmother one night, "I'm never going to be able to have a life now. Nobody will ever want to date me. Look at me - I'm a mess."

When he came to see me, it was about two years later. His other injuries had healed, but he was still missing many teeth, and the few he had remaining were chipped or broken. In short, his mouth was an absolute mess.

We extracted all of his teeth and did a full dental restoration with implants, top and bottom, and we were able to give him one of the most beautiful smiles you've ever seen. When we finished up, this kid was very grateful and very happy. His grandmother, the person who brought him to most his appointments with us, told me about him thinking that he'd never even have a chance at having a wife and family. Now, with his gorgeous new smile, he's dating all the time. And instead of being withdrawn and depressed, he has fantastic self-confidence.

That's just one example of how restoring a great smile can change someone's whole outlook on life.

THE DEVELOPMENT OF DENTAL IMPLANTS

A dental implant is a titanium fixture that is placed, or "implanted", in a person's jaw bone, where it serves a similar function as the root of a natural tooth. The implant acts as an anchor to hold a crown or some other kind of a dental prosthetic, such as a bridge or denture. Implants can be used to replace anything from a single missing tooth to an entire set of teeth.

There's actually evidence of something like dental implants being used around 4,000 years ago. There have been remains found in China of people with bamboo pegs that had been tapped into their bones, and some Egyptian mummies have teeth made of ivory. But the history of modern-day dental implants goes back to 1952, when an orthopedic surgeon in Sweden, Dr. Branemark, discovered that titanium implants adhered extremely well to bone. A few years after that, Dr. Leonard Linkow placed the first dental implant into a jaw bone. The Branemark System, developed in 1965, is still the basis for dental implant treatment.

There have been a lot of different styles of implants used over the years, such as a blade implant that was screwed into the jaw. Some doctors have used subperiosteal implants, where a metal frame is attached to the jaw. There was something called zygoma implants that go through the sinus and up into the zygomatic arch.

The dental implants being used today are "root form" implants. Root form implants are very versatile in the ways they can be used, and they're smaller in diameter than many previous types of implants, making them easier to place. Implants have been in use for over 50 years, and they've proven to be a safe and effective dental treatment. They've gotten better and better over the years, and the implant process is continually being improved.

Dental implants are the ideal treatment option for replacing missing teeth, because they save tooth structure (EXAMPLE: If a patient is missing one tooth an implant can be placed. The teeth on either side of the missing tooth do not have to be cut down to do a bridge, you don't have to damage two good teeth to put one tooth back). They are also ideal treatment for missing teeth because they can eliminate the need for having a denture that comes in and out. Implants are placed with fixed prosthetics such as crowns so that a patient has a full set of teeth permanently fixed in place.

IMPLANT TECHNOLOGY

The technology for doing implants has advanced significantly. When I first started placing implants, we didn't have the excellent surgical guides that we have now that are so helpful in terms of getting the exact right placement for an implant.

Dental CAT scans using cone beam technology, or CBCT, are one of the most important technological advances. CBCT gives the dentist or oral surgeon a digital scan of the patient's teeth and surrounding tissue and bone structure. That provides a 3D image showing what volume of bone a patient has, how thick the bone is, and exactly where the nerves are so that we can avoid damaging those.

The biggest risk in doing implants has always been the possibility of hitting a nerve and damaging it, potentially causing permanent numbness around that area. This is what has the majority of General Dentists in America afraid to place implants. But with the advanced technology we have now, that danger has been virtually eliminated.

Doctors are able to make precise digital measurements of everything, pre-plan the implant placement, and then export that information to a 3D printer and produce a surgical guide that is laid right in the patient's mouth to guide the doctor in doing the implant placement surgery.

THE RISKS OF NOT GETTING IMPLANTS

I mentioned the main risk associated with getting implants – nerve damage – and the fact that it's pretty much been eliminated. The truly severe risks are those that result from *not* getting implants when they're needed, when people are missing one or more teeth. When missing teeth aren't replaced, over time there is significant bone loss in the jaw. It turns into a slippery slope where people end up with more missing teeth and more and more bone loss. That affects both your health and your appearance. Some patients think it's just one missing tooth. No big deal, I can eat without it. What they do not understand is that one can bite with 250-300 lbs of pressure. The teeth all work together.

Therefore a single missing tooth is a big concern. Often times an unreplaced missing tooth means 4 missing teeth with time.

Bone loss in the jaw not only changes the look of person's face - it also leads to increasing misalignment of the remaining teeth and to them becoming loose in the jaw and more prone to falling out. Your remaining teeth begin to shift and extrude, which means they push up higher out of the gum. The remaining teeth appear to get longer. They haven't really gotten longer; it's just that more of the tooth is showing above the gum line. That's where the expression about looking "long in the tooth" comes from. The teeth pushing up like means that they become looser in a person's mouth, because they're less well-attached to the jaw bone. That, of course, eventually leads to losing more teeth.

WHY IMPLANTS ARE A BETTER TREATMENT THAN DENTURES

Dentures don't effectively solve the problem because dentures won't stop the bone loss from occurring. Even if you just have one tooth missing, it's best to get an implant placed as soon as possible, because that's the only treatment that effectively prevents bone loss in the jaw. Getting an implant not only restores the proper function of chewing and a good cosmetic look – it also keeps the other teeth from shifting and starting to come loose.

There are a lot of significant general health issues related to missing teeth. When you have several missing teeth, it can actually reduce your natural lifespan by up to 10 years. One reason for that is because not having all your teeth makes it difficult to eat the different foods that you need for proper nutrition. Certain foods that people with missing teeth have trouble eating are some of the most important sources of good nutrition, such as raw fruits and vegetables.

You're also more likely to have to take medicine – 38% more likely, in fact – to deal with some of the health issues that arise from missing teeth. People sometimes have to take medicine to help them digest their food properly. A lot of people with missing teeth end up taking antidepressants. When people don't feel good about their smile, a major part of their appearance, they become depressed because they feel self-conscious and have a poor self-image. They feel embarrassed when they're out in public, and usually their whole social life suffers.

Dentures aren't really a good fix for those self-esteem issues, because with dentures people are always worried about the possible embarrassment of having their teeth fall out while they're eating, or even while they're just talking to someone. Getting dental implants helps you stay looking young. A patient with all their teeth can chew with about 250 to 300 pounds of pressure, but a patient with full dentures is often chewing with as little as 30 pounds of pressure – only about 10% of what's natural. In addition to the bone loss that results from missing teeth, the jaw muscles become weaker, and those things combined change the appearance of your face so that you look much older than you actually are. Many have the appearance that their face has caved in.

TREATMENT WITH DENTAL IMPLANTS

The treatment time required for placing implants and then the prosthetics, such as crowns or dentures that attach to them, varies depending on the individual patient and on exactly how much work is being done.

You schedule a consultation for an exam to make a diagnosis and come up with a treatment plan. Then you come back for the placement of the implant. Ordinarily, a dentist will then wait three to six months for the implant to properly integrate with the bone. Then the patient comes back and the dentist gets an impression for the dental prosthetic. A dental lab or the dentist makes the prosthetic, and then the dentist places that during a final visit.

Full reconstruction cases require a few more appointments. However, the technology for doing implants has become so advanced now that in some cases we can actually bring someone in, extract all their remaining teeth, place implants, and put a beautiful prosthetic on top of that, all in one visit. We'll have another follow-up visit three to six months later, but they can walk out in one day with a beautiful smile. Of course, it's not quite that simple. In order to be able to do that, you have to do a little bit of preparation work first.

DIAGNOSIS, TREATMENT PLAN, AND PLACEMENT

It's important for the dentist to start off right with a proper diagnosis and treatment plan. The technology we have now enables dentists to go beyond using traditional x-rays and get actual 3D images of the patient's teeth and surrounding bone structure. I can actually do a virtual placement of the implants in a computer program, working from a dental CAT scan, and then create the surgical guide that's placed right in the patient's mouth to precisely guide me in placing the implants. I have drills with a depth stop on them that guide me at the right angle and depth at every step in the placement process, making implant placement a procedure that I can do very quickly and safely for the patient.

Part of the diagnosis involves the dentist checking to see how much bone there is in the jaw in terms of width and height, and checking for adequate space. We don't want to run the implant into an adjacent natural tooth, so we need to make sure we have adequate space. It's also important to make sure there's a sufficient amount of distance between the implant and nerves, because we don't want to injure any nerves when placing the implant. If there's not enough width or height, then the dentist has to consider a bone graft. That may mean raising the sinus or building the bone up to be taller and or wider.

The average patient, once they hear implants, may get a little scared and go, "My gosh, you're going to screw something into my bone." But the fact is that there are very few nerve endings in the bone, so there's usually very little discomfort. Getting an implant is actually pretty easy. In fact, there's usually less pain from getting an implant than there is from having a couple of regular fillings done.

The dentist ordinarily places a temporary on top of the implant when the implant surgery is done. The dentist or oral surgeon checks to see if the implant is stable, which means it can be torqued to 35 N/cm (Newton centimeters) of torque without it moving. If the bone is softer, so that it doesn't torque out sufficiently without moving, then you may have to wait 6 months rather than 3 months to restore it. In cases like that, the dentist doesn't put a regular temporary on but places a little piece that's called a healing cap. The healing cap allows the tissue surrounding the implant to form a good, solid seal around it. A different type of temporary is then made.

Then we typically wait three to six months for the implant to integrate properly with the bone. The waiting period is for new bone growth to occur around the threads of the implant. We want new bone to grow inside of, and all the way around, the threads of the implant screw. Three months is usually a sufficient time frame for that to occur. You may have to wait a bit longer for integration to take place if the bone quality is softer.

TEMPORARY TO PERMANENT PROSTHETIC

After sufficient integration with the jaw bone, the patient comes back to get an impression for making the permanent crown. The dentist just unscrews the temporary piece and screws in a piece to make an impression. It's a quick and easy process that doesn't require numbing the patient.

In getting an impression, we can either use the traditional "goop" material in a dental tray, or with the technology that we have now, we can do a digital impression using a computer program. The digital impression works especially well if the space around the implant is kind of tight, making it difficult to get a firm impression using gel and trays. Either way, we get an impression and then either send the impression to a dental lab, or we can actually make the crowns right in our office with ceramic metal composites.

When the permanent crown or other prosthetic is ready, we place a small piece that's called an abutment. The abutment is screwed into the implant and used to support the crown, bridge, or denture. We torque the abutment firmly into place with a little torque wrench, and then we place the crown, bridge, or denture on top of the abutment, and the patient has a beautiful, natural-looking smile, and their teeth and jaws function properly. If you want to picture it in your mind, from the bottom to the top you've got the implant, the abutment, and then the crown or other prosthetic.

HOW LONG DO DENTAL IMPLANTS LAST?

Dental implants offer a good, long-term solution for dental problems because they usually last longer than many other dental treatments. Studies have shown that at the 10-year mark, 95% of implants are still in place and going strong. Actually, if an implant is going to fail, that most often happens within the first year. The prosthetics that go on top of the implant are usually good for about 10 to 15 years. A lot of times a dentist may have to replace the crown but not the actual implant.

An implant can fail for a number of reasons. It might fail due the way it was placed. An implant can also fail as a result of general health problems, or because medicine the patient is taking causes the bone to weaken. Smoking can cause problems with how long implants last. The failure rate at the 10-year mark for smokers is twice as high as the failure rate for implants in non-smokers.

The most common cause of implant failure is bite problems. When we do implants, it's critical to get the bite right. Patients with implants need to make sure they go in for regular dental visits every six months and have their bite checked at least annually. That's important because the bite can shift a little bit over time. But as long as the dentist notices the change before any damage has resulted from the bite shift, then he can make the necessary adjustments and avoid any serious problems.

MAINTENANCE OF IMPLANTS

Just as with any dental restoration, it's important to take good care of your dental implants after you receive them. It's not difficult to take good care of implants – you just brush and floss like you would with natural teeth. I think it's also very important to use a Water Pik type of tooth cleaning tool. That helps keep your restorations really clean and your gums healthy.

As long as you practice good dental hygiene and go in for regular dental visits every six months to get your bite checked and get a professional cleaning, then you can expect your implants to last a very long time. I have patients with implants up to nineteen years – which is as long as I've been doing implants – that are still going strong.

WHEN ARE IMPLANTS NOT AN APPROPRIATE TREATMENT OPTION?

There are some situations where implants are not an appropriate treatment option. People with serious health issues may not be good candidates for implants, especially people with severe autoimmune diseases. People who are taking IV bisphosphonate drugs (a group of drugs that inhibit bone resorption and are used for treating diseases like osteoporosis) shouldn't get implants because that type of medication can cause severe problems with getting implants. Most uncontrolled diabetics are not usually good candidates for implants, although I have personally done implants for patients with uncontrolled diabetes and had good results and everything was fine – but it's still considered a big risk.

An alternative treatment for someone just missing one or two teeth could be doing a dental bridge. A bridge is a dental prosthetic that attaches to a person's natural teeth adjacent to the missing teeth.

I don't generally like using dentures, but sometimes that is the best treatment option for someone who can't get implants. I think the best use of dentures is when they're implant-supported. But in a case where someone just cannot get implants and a bridge won't be sufficient, then treatment with dentures is certainly better than not treating the problem at all.

Fortunately, most patients can have implants. Even if they've suffered some bone loss in their jaw, they may still be able to get implants done with the help of getting some bone grafting first. A lot of cases require some bone grafting. I had a patient just the other day – Her sinus had dropped down to the point where she didn't have enough height to allow for implants. Also, her bone width was very narrow – wide enough to allow the implants to be placed but not wide enough to give them proper support. We raised her sinus, built more bone width, and placed the implants all at the same time. Sometimes we might have to do one part of that and then wait a few weeks or months before doing the next part.

If you lose a tooth or multiple teeth, it's best for you to get to an implant dentist as soon as possible, so that you can get implants placed before you lose much bone. Let me share a statistic with you: If you had all your teeth extracted and then waited one year before getting implants, during just that one year you would lose 25% of the width and 4 mm of height in your jaw bone. That's why it's really important to seek treatment for missing teeth right away.

THE COST FOR IMPLANT TREATMENT

The cost of getting dental implants varies widely, depending on a number of factors. Some of the primary factors that affect cost include the following:

1. The number of implants being placed

2. The brand or quality of the implants being placed

3. The type of dental prosthetic being attached to the implant

4. The dental lab costs

5. What area of the country you're in

6. The amount of bone grafting necessary

Implant treatment can range in cost anywhere from around $3,500 up to as much as $100,000. That's obviously a very, very wide range of potential costs. I'd estimate that the typical cost for a single implant is somewhere around four thousand dollars. To do a traditional full restoration with complete upper and lower implants replacing all your natural teeth, the average cost is approximately $85,000. To do upper and lower all on 4 the typical cost is $48,000 – $60,000.

Dental insurance doesn't usually cover implants, although I have seen that changing in recent years. There are more insurance plans now that will pay at least part of the cost of getting implants. But the total cost for an implant is almost always going to exceed the maximum cap of dental insurance plans – the most they'll pay out in one calendar year. So even with a very good dental insurance plan, patients are still looking at a significant out-of-pocket expense for getting implants. Of course, dentists recognize that fact and so most dental practices that offer implant treatment are also willing to help patients out with financing or payment plans. That way you don't have to come up with the total amount all at once.

I tell patients this: Whether you have insurance coverage or not, the overall health benefits of getting dental implants far outweigh the financial costs. I wouldn't let the insurance issue determine whether or not I got an implant. Because of the serious health issues that can be caused by missing teeth – I'm talking about both your oral health and your overall physical health – choosing to *not* get implants could easily end up costing you a lot more in total medical expenses in the long run than the cost of implants.

COSMETIC BENEFITS OF IMPLANTS

As far as cosmetic issues, implants are an ideal treatment to restore or create a really beautiful smile for someone who's lost a tooth or multiple teeth, or who needs to have all of their teeth replaced.

I do a lot of cosmetic dentistry with implants. If someone is missing one or more teeth, and they want to get an ideal smile, there are a lot of cosmetic options we can use with crowns, veneers, hybrids or dentures. In many cases, you really can't tell by looking which teeth are implants with crowns, which teeth have had veneers applied, and which teeth are the person's natural teeth. It's possible for a dentist to match the color of adjacent teeth with implant prosthetics. And if a patient is having a full upper and lower restoration done with implants, we can basically make them any color they want.

It's no secret that most patients who spend the money for complete replacement of all their teeth with implants usually want that bright, million dollar, movie star kind of perfect smile – and we can certainly give it to them.

FINDING THE BEST DENTIST TO DO YOUR IMPLANTS

Dental implants represent a substantial investment in your dental health, your overall health, and your appearance. Therefore, you obviously want to get your implants done by a highly-qualified, highly-skilled, and experienced dentist.

There aren't a lot of specific requirements from dental boards in terms of how many classes you have to take or what level of training a dentist has to have in order to do implants. Because of that, it's important that you, as the patient, do the necessary research to find a really highly-trained and skilled dentist to place your implants.

There is a lot in play with regards to the skill of the person doing the procedure. You have to keep the bone cool while doing the implant placement and that takes skill that's developed with experience. If a dentist mistakenly places an implant into an infected site, then you're going to lose it. It's important to make sure there's no infection where implants are being placed. And of course the dentist has to place the implant properly and make sure the bite is just right. There's definitely significant skill required for doing implants.

IMPLANT PLACEMENT EDUCATION AND TRAINING

I can tell you that in my own training, I initially went and took a two-day training course, and the next week I placed my first 3 implants. My Grandfather received implants number 2 and 3 (they last him the rest of his life). I quickly realized that I needed to learn a lot more and get more training in order to be able to do the kind of top-notch, high-quality work that would guarantee my patients the best possible results. I realized that I did not know how to build height or width. I didn't know how to graft the sinus. There were so many patients I still could not help. I had to get more education and more information.

I studied for quite some time at the Misch International Implant Institute. Dr. Misch spent his career on improving dental implant dentistry, and he developed many of the principles and classifications that have since become standard in modern implant dentistry. The Institute offers a full range of courses in dental implant surgery and in creating and placing the dental restorations that are attached to implants. Studying at the Misch

Institute was terrific – I learned a lot and got a lot of hands-on experience.

And I didn't stop there. I continued to seek out more education and training all over the United States and around the world. It's important for dentists to continue learning, continue taking classes and getting advanced training because the technology is constantly changing and improving, and you have to keep up with that if you want to offer patients the best possible treatment experience and results.

By 2006 I had so much education and training and gained so much experience in doing implants, that I was asked by the largest dental supply company in the world to teach other dentists to place and restore dental implants. We signed contracts and since 2007 I've been teaching implant dentistry to other dentists. I've trained well over 1,000 dentists, hands-on, in placing implants and doing implant restorations. I've trained hundreds of dentists in procedures such as bone and sinus grafting.

When you're looking into getting dental implants, don't be afraid to ask questions. Ask the dentist about his training and experience. Ask to see some "before and after" photos of patients he's done implant dentistry on. Most dentists who have made the effort to become an expert in doing implant dentistry and do a lot of implant treatment, will have a lot of those "before and after" pictures. They'll also usually have their training certificates displayed in their office because they're quite naturally proud of having undertaken extensive advanced training.

You can also ask if they have a former implant patient you can contact. You can ask the other team members in the dental practice questions. They'll know what kind of treatments the doctor does a lot of and has a high degree of skill in doing.

Most dentists will honestly tell you about the level of their education, training, and experience in implant dentistry. Earlier in my practice, when I first began doing implant dentistry, I would tell patients right up front that I didn't have much experience yet in doing implants, but that I was continually getting more training, education, and practice, and that I was focusing my dental practice specifically on doing comprehensive implant and cosmetic dentistry. That way they knew that I was dedicated to becoming very highly-skilled in doing implant treatments.

CHANGING PEOPLE'S LIVES WITH IMPLANT DENTISTRY

As I've already said, implant dentistry is the best treatment option for people with missing teeth. A skilled and well-trained dentist can give you remarkable cosmetic results with implant dentistry.

I had a lady named Rose who came to see me, a very nice lady in her 70's. She told me right up front that the reason she'd come to see me was because she couldn't eat. She was losing weight but just couldn't eat. Her problem stemmed from the fact that she had several missing teeth, and she just couldn't chew food properly. We discussed some treatment options I could offer her with dental implants.

I remember it was interesting when we discussed the cost. I vividly remember her saying, "Well, that's a lot of money, but I have the money. I just really need to decide whether it's worth it or not."

We talked some more – I answered her questions – and she finally decided to go ahead with implants. I was glad that she did, because her missing teeth were severely threatening her overall health. It's pretty alarming when someone says they can't eat.

Once we placed her implants with restorations, she started getting back to a more healthy weight almost immediately. She didn't gain too much weight – she just got back to being at a healthy weight, and she looked much better. She looked healthier and she also looked significantly more attractive. The implants made a tremendously positive change in her appearance – not to mention enabling her to eat all the foods she'd been missing. Her energy level was much higher.

There are two things I wanted to share about Rose's case. One of them is about my dental assistant who worked with me on doing Rose's implants. She happened to run into Rose out at a restaurant, and Rose called her over to her table. Rose asked my assistant, "Do you remember what I said I wanted to eat more than anything in the world once I could eat again?" My assistant did remember, and so she said, "Yes, I remember that you said you wanted to eat salad." Rose smiled and said, "That's right", and she stuck her fork into a piece of lettuce, lifted it up to her mouth, and proceeded to enjoy eating it. She proudly declared, "I can eat anything I want to now, and it's wonderful."

The second thing I wanted to share about this case occurred about nine and a half years later. We got a phone call at the office, and the person calling asked to speak with that same dental assistant. When she got on the phone, the person calling said to her, "On behalf of our whole family, we just wanted to thank you and Dr. Eggleston for helping Rose with getting those dental implants. This is the first phone call that we've made after informing other family members that Rose passed away today. Anyway, we wanted to call and thank you because we believe that getting those implants enabled her to live another nine and a half years. I don't know if Rose ever told you this, but at the time she came to see you, she was losing weight so fast that her doctor told us that she was dying. You gave her an extra nine and half years of really enjoying her life. "

When I teach implant dentistry courses to other dentists around the country, I often tell this story. Even though I've told it many times, it still often brings tears to my eyes. Anyway, I tell that story to other doctors I'm teaching, and then I ask them a question: What if I had chickened out and not offered her the implant treatment – the treatment that she really needed - just because it was expensive and I was afraid of her getting upset about the cost? If I'd done that, I might have robbed her and her family of nine and a half happy years together – robbed her of nine and a half years of her life.

My point in telling dentists that story is just to illustrate for them very clearly the fact that we need to avoid making money issues the focus of decisions about treatment. Instead, we need to make sure that our primary concern is what's best for the patient. We always need to ask ourselves, "What's the best treatment plan for the patient, what would I do if this was my mouth and health – totally apart from cost issues?" That's also a good story to help remind us not to try to make decisions for patients on our own. Instead, we need to help our patients make their own decisions, their own choices about treatment options. Our job is to apply that treatment option to the very best of our ability, so that we make sure that our patients end up with the best possible result, the kind of result that gives them health, the look they want and that helps them smile confidently and feel good about themselves. That's my aim when I go to work every single day.

ABOUT JIM EGGLESTON, DDS

Eggleston Dental Care
www.EgglestonDentalCare.com

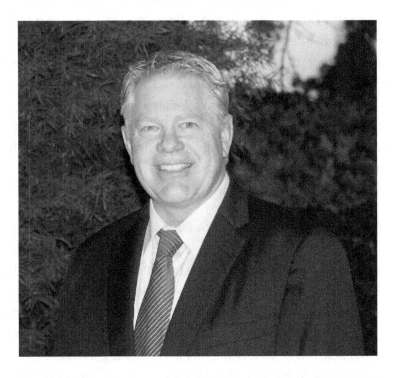

Dr. Jim Eggleston is a Turlock-based professional who has more than 20 years of experience as a cosmetic and implant dentist. Dr. Eggleston's dedication to helping patients obtain the perfect smile has made him a trusted professional among his patients. A 1992 graduate of University of the Pacific in San Francisco, Dr. Eggleston has spent thousands of hours in continuing education to insure that he remains abreast of the latest developments in all areas of dentistry.

Dr. Eggleston is a recipient of the Mastership with the Intentional Congress of Oral Implantology, and is a member of the American Dental Association, California Dental Association,

Stanislaus Dental Foundation, Academy of Cosmetic Dentistry and the Crown Council.

According to Dr. Eggleston, "When I began my dental career, I knew I wanted to offer my patient's state of the art dentistry, the best dental care available. I wanted to be able to offer the healthiest treatment available, and I wanted the opportunity to change the lives of my patients. I have worked long and hard to achieve the degrees, certificates, and create a lecturing field, but it still comes down to this: the feeling I get when I see someone cry the moment they see their new smile, the feeling I get when I see the renewed confidence and self-esteem that has been given back to a patient, and the feeling I get knowing I can in many cases extend a grandparent's life up to 10 years, giving them 10 more years to celebrate life with other loved ones." This is what motivates me to continue learning and teaching. These results and feelings cannot be purchased. What I have learned is as I do the kind of dentistry that changes people's lives, the life that is changed the most is mine.

Dr. Eggleston has provided hands-on training to more than 1,000 dentists in placing and restoring implants, and has trained hundreds of other professionals in bone and sinus grafting. In his extensive training of dentists since 2007, he has trained hundreds of auxiliary team members in various dental services, helping them to provide top-quality dental care to their patients. Dr. Eggleston proudly supports dental professionals in becoming the best providers of care possible.

LEADING THE WAY WITH DIGITAL DENTISTRY

The field of cosmetic dentistry is experiencing a major digital boom, thanks to all of the technological advances that are continually being made. Digital dentistry, in the simplest terms, refers to the use of digital, computerized technology in place of traditional techniques that have typically been used for dental procedures in the past. These new treatment methods and techniques are ever increasing in their scope and the opportunities they present to dentists and doctors around the world, helping to dramatically reduce or eliminate issues that may occur because of human error or inability to complete procedures and treatments with the most ideal results.

Dentistry is still partially a form of art, as well as a skill, so the human element is still absolutely necessary; human skill and vision is a predominant aspect of dentistry that allows patients to have the most stable and beautiful smiles. The digital aspect being brought in to dentistry is there to help dentists and doctors elevate their abilities and give their patients the smile of their dreams.

New Technology and Its Benefits

In my practice the biggest change in terms of digital dentistry is the addition of Cone Beam CT technology. This is a newer technology but one that is spreading rapidly throughout many dental offices. Within surgical care, this technology has become almost a standard of care. Cone Beam CT scanners differ from traditional CT scanners in that they capture images more quickly and use a much lower level of radiation.

Both Cone Beam CT scanners and traditional scanners fall into the tomography category of technology, however, the Cone Beam scanners are able to capture the information in one pass (less radiation) – versus a rotating x-ray tube used by traditional scanners which requires overlap of the slices. This new type of scan is a major improvement because it provides the dentist with a three-dimensional view of what's going on under the skin in the patient's mouth and jaw in an office setting. This enables the dentist to have a better understanding of exactly what they're dealing with when treating patients, especially when surgical or more invasive procedures are necessary.

Prior to the use of CT scans – especially the Cone Beam scanner - dentists and oral surgeons relied on traditional flat film, radiography - x-rays. These help to a point, but they don't provide a full image of the patient's condition. With only a two-dimensional image to work with dentists had to try to interpret – rather than precisely knowing – what was going on in a patient's mouth, jaw, and head. The major downside with flat films this is that while we often had correct interpretations of the condition, there were also times when we didn't. The Cone Beam scanner offers us the ability to be much more accurate in treating patients because it provides more clear and detailed information.

Here is a great example I just had when writing this chapter:

Karen is a 73 years old female patient who arrived to her general dentist with a complaint that her crown (that was placed by another dentist) keeps falling off. After careful inspection, the general dentist noted that there was not enough tooth structure to properly restore the tooth. He replaced the crown with temporary cement and sent her to my office.

Pre-operative x-ray given to me from her general dentist are shown on the left (note that the root canal). The patient was interested in getting an implant so we took a CT scan of the tooth to evaluate the bone quality (see that image on the right).

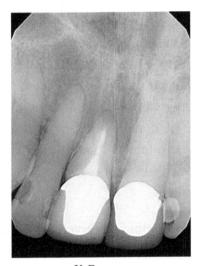 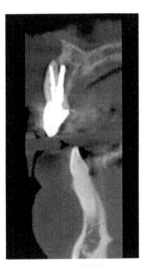

X-Ray   Cone Beam CT Scan

This CT scan shows that the root canal was completed correctly, but when it was restored with a post and core there were issues. The alternate view provided with this digital technology demonstrated that the post was placed outside the tooth and over time led to destruction of the bone behind the tooth. Without this bone an attempted immediate implant would

*have failed. Without the CBCT I would failed the patient and that
is just another example of why I choose to be on the leading edge
of digital dentistry.*

MORE ABOUT CONE BEAM TECHNOLOGY

I'd like to delve a little further into how Cone Beam technology
works and how it helps me – and any dentist or surgeon using it
– to better treat patients.

As I mentioned previously, using Cone Beam technology is an
important part of helping dentists and oral surgeons plan and
execute surgeries in the most effective way possible. Using the
images provided by the scans, they can visualize the surgery and
actually conduct a practice surgery on the computer. They are
able to see things better such as the patient's bone density, tooth
positions, and the patient's anatomy when it comes to things like
nerve or sinus location, bone quality, and space needed for
implants. Virtually doing the surgery before actually touching the
patient, planning what needs to be done, as well as determining
the best ways to accomplish these things ahead of time, makes it
much easier to do the actual surgery in the best manner possible
and get the best result for the patient.

Unfortunately, Cone Beam technology isn't yet a standard in
every dentist's office. It's one of the newer technologies available.
Fortunately, it is rapidly growing in use, especially among oral
surgeons, orthodontists, endodontists, and periodontists.

TRADITIONAL IMPRESSIONS

Before I can talk about digital impressions I think it's important
to explain what traditional impressions are to help you compare
and contrast the two. Prior to the creation of digital impressions,
dentists were – and still are, in many offices – using alginate-or

THE MILLION DOLLAR SMILE

vinylpoly siloxane (big words that describe the type of materials used) impressions. Basically, these materials start as a gooey liquid and are put into a tray that is then inserted into the patient's mouth. The materials then begin to harden, making an impression of the patient's teeth. Before the materials dry entirely, the tray is removed from the patient's mouth and set out to become completely hard. Afterward, a stony material is then poured into the impression to create a solid, physical model of the patient's teeth.

There are considerable disadvantages to this method of creating impressions. Each of the materials used to create these impressions has different expansion and contraction rates, meaning they can shrink or expand. They are very sensitive to humidity and environmental temperatures. Any or all of those factors can affect how the model accuracy when compared to the patient's teeth ends up being.

Another one of the major disadvantages of the traditional impression method is how patients react to these impressions. Most don't like the sensation of the gooey material in their mouth, the size of the tray used to hold the material, and how difficult it can be to remove the tray once the material starts to harden. Some patients have a significant gag reflex or a sensation of not being able to breathe enough.

Along with this, the time it takes to let the material set is sometimes irritating for patients and can set back what we accomplish during an appointment. If anything goes wrong with taking the impression, such as improper placement, a bad fit, or if the patient moves, then the impression has to be redone. This takes even more time, and, it's more costly. (A quick side note: it takes about $30 to $50 to get a good upper and lower impression. If we have to redo them, that's more money.) One of my goals is always to cut down on the amount of time the patient has to sit in the chair. It decreases any anxiety they have and increases our productivity. It can also help cut down on cost using a digitally based impression technique.

A final disadvantage to mention is the potential for breaking the impressions. Once the physical impression has been made, if they are dropped, moved, or taken out of the mold too forcefully, they can break. Once they're broken, they can't be used, because gluing them back together doesn't generally provide an accurate enough reflection of the patient's teeth to make a good restoration.

DIGITAL IMPRESSIONS

Now that we've covered traditional impressions, let's talk about digital impressions. In my practice, we use an intraoral scanner. It's a key element in how we operate and function. It has drastically cut down on inaccurate impressions and is less stressful for our patients. We are able to avoid subjecting patient to gooey materials and trays, and because the impression is digital, there's no fear of breaking, damaging, or losing them. Also, it takes less time for my staff to take an intraoral scan, which means the appointment progresses more quickly, we can get more done, and it takes less time out of the patient's day. We can also see the impressions in real time, so if there is any inaccuracy – or we need a clearer picture – we can immediately retake the scan while the patient is still in the chair.

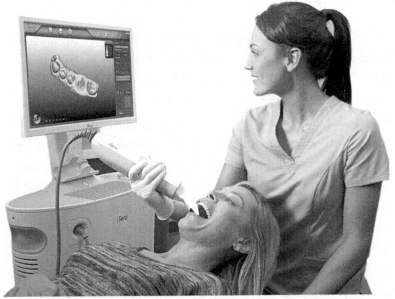

Intraoral scanning of patient.
Safe, easier on the patient, and more accurate than traditional methods.

Another huge benefit is that because the impressions are electronic, we can send the file to the lab much more quickly than the physical stone impressions can be transported. This decreases turnaround time in processing the impressions and moves the patient's case along more quickly.

Finally, one of the biggest advantages that I've witnessed is the fact that intraoral scans can be saved indefinitely without using up any physical space. This means that, for example, if we create a denture for someone using their digital impression and the denture breaks, we can then use the impressions to create a new denture for them without having to redo the impressions. This saves an incredible amount of work and time, cuts out the need for the patient to come back in, and it's a huge money saver as well.

CAD/CAM MILLING AND CEREC

CAD/CAM (computer-aided design/computer-aided manufacturing) milling technology, especially the E4D or CEREC system – which is a CAD/CAM product – is becoming more and more popular in dental offices. In some instances, it enables dentists to do chair-side milling of crowns and smaller bridges. Utilizing this technology, we can create the restorations that patients need in one sitting. This is incredibly useful because it decreases turnaround time drastically. Traditional methods – namely creating all restorations in a lab – can take two to three weeks. At most, using the CAD/CAM technology lets us create what we need in less than a week, but, sometimes, as I said above, we can make them almost instantly. It really depends on what the patient wants and needs. Regardless, the time difference is remarkable.

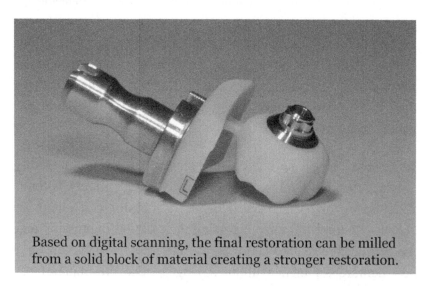

Based on digital scanning, the final restoration can be milled from a solid block of material creating a stronger restoration.

Also, like with Cone Beam and intraoral scans, this technology improves how we predict the outcomes of our treatment plan and decreases our margin of error significantly. For example, using something like the E4D or CEREC system, dentists can more accurately narrow the edge around where we connect a crown to a patient's tooth, meaning it fits better, functions better, and is less likely to come loose or fall out. It also means that we can decrease the amount of metal, porcelain or various materials used. This improves the aesthetic outcome for the patient.

VIRTUAL SURGERY

Before the advent of digitally guided or virtual surgery, we used traditional 2D x-rays and essentially eyeballed, for example, an implant against the x-ray, saying, "This seems about the right size." We didn't have a true understanding of the full, 3D volumetric of the patient's anatomy in general and specifically around where the implant would be placed. We had to go into surgery and explore placement once we were directly working on the patient. This often led to errors in sizing, positioning – either from a depth, orientation, or an angulation perspective, meaning the angle at which the implant needed to be placed. Although virtual surgery is advancing rapidly in the dental field, as recently as 2015 less than 1% of implant surgery cases were virtually guided, meaning, there is a lot of room for error and more patients who got less than the very best results.

Virtual surgery allows us to harness the advantages of digital dentistry, expanding what we know about patients and their specific needs by using Cone Beam scans and intraoral scans as guides. This enables us to improve patient outcomes by planning beforehand, making a virtual model of our patients and mapping out precisely what needs to be done, and how, before we begin operating. It's much more controlled, which means it leads to a less stressful and unknown operation for us and better results for our patients.

In my own practice, currently more than 95% of my cases are virtually guided. With each one of my patients, I take a CT scan and I use that in conjunction with an intraoral scan. This gives me a clear virtual representation of my patient that I can reference once the patient has left the chair. I can work at my desk and plan out exactly where I need to place an implant, making me confident that the depth, orientation, and angle is perfect before I actually place the implant. This technology also enables us to explore the patient's soft and hard tissue – the gums and jaw bones – helping to determine if changes to the tissue need to be made before operating. Ultimately, when I go into surgery, I'm as confident as possible, knowing that I've used all the technology available to assist me in operating and giving my patient that best result possible.

Using virtual guides also helps cut down on the time it takes to perform oral surgery. The majority of the decisions that need to be made are done beforehand using the virtual model we've created. The virtual guide directs the oral surgeon, allowing them to follow the surgical plan already created and practiced on a computer. This is great for the oral surgeon and also for the patient. It cuts down on the time the patient spends under anesthesia, taking less of a toll on their body and helping them to recover more quickly.

ON THE SUBJECT OF ANESTHESIA

Since I was just talking about it, I'd like to mention a new digital advancement when it comes to anesthesia. There are now anesthesia machines available that can distribute the proper medications based on the length of time a patient needs to be anesthetized, their body weight, and other factors, using an infusion pump. I utilize these machines which are specifically helpful for surgeries that take a longer amount of time.

These pumps make it easier and safer to get patients to a steady level of anesthetization and keep them there for hours at a time if needed, without using any more medication than is necessary. This means that they don't fluctuate up and down in terms of consciousness. It's much better for the patient because it keeps their heart rate and blood pressure at a safe, steady level. They're comfortable throughout the procedure, not restless, making it easier for the surgeon to do what needs to be done. Additionally, the medications we are able to use are less stressful on the patient, resulting in less post-operative side effects such as nausea and allowing them to come out from the anesthesia quicker and recover faster. In many cases, I'm able to discharge patients within 15 minutes even after a three or four-hour surgery.

A DENTAL SUCCESS STORY

I'd like to share the story of one of my patients here. It presents a real-world example and paints a great picture of how digital dentistry can transform the effectiveness of patient treatment.

I had a gentleman come to see me. He needed a full mouth extraction. At 89 years old, he had a compromised medical history. We had a few anesthetic options, but doing local anesthesia wasn't the best choice given his history of anxiety. We could also have sent him to the operating room for general anesthesia, however, this option would have involved going to the hospital and would be harder for him to recover from, especially considering his age and compromised medical status. He decided – and I agreed – that the best option was to use conscious sedation – sometimes referred to as 'twilight' sedation – in the clinic where we had a machine that delivered a consistent, controlled level of medication to keep him calm and comfortable.

We were able to remove all of his upper and lower teeth, reshape his bone, and place a total of 10 implants in less than three hours. Under traditional circumstances, this procedure would take at least four hours or more. I was able to successfully remove his teeth and replace them with implants because I'd planned his entire treatment virtually, utilizing the Cone Beam CT scans and intraoral scans. Because of digital dentistry, we were able to give him his smile back, using the safest sedation option, in a minimal amount of time.

DIGITAL DENTISTRY IN ORTHODONTICS

Digital dentistry is playing a major role in orthodontics. I work with a number of orthodontists who are utilizing intraoral scans and various digital programs to help plan where their patients' teeth need to end up, how they need to move, how quickly they can be moved, and to assist in planning the techniques that will help them accomplish the best outcome for the patients. There are some advanced digital programs that can be used with machines that bend the wires used in braces.

Other digital technologies they use help them plan where the brackets and bands need to go and how they need to be placed, and then the specially-crafted wire is inserted. The orthodontist then already knows that the force the wire places on the teeth, teamed with the brackets and bands, is going to move the teeth at the right speed and get them into the right position because he's used virtual models ahead of time. This cuts down significantly on the time it takes to put the braces on, make the needed changes during each phase of movement, and it can ultimately help cut down on the length of time the patient is in the chair per appointment and the total length of treatment time the braces need to stay on. Many orthodontists I work closely with are also utilizing 3D printers to print up models of the patient's teeth at each stage of the treatment plan, enabling them to make guides and trays for patients to utilize in between the stages to keep the teeth where they need to be.

The newer trend in orthodontics is to virtually plan the the tooth movements. Then break the desired movements into steps that is tolerable for the biology of the human body to accept. These steps are then printed into clear retainers that the patient sequentially wears over several months to achieve the desired movement. This process works well and is becoming the go to option for people who do not want traditional brackets and wires. In my opinion it is critical that before the patient begins a trained orthodontist still physically sees the patient to ensure that this is the correct treatment.

3D PRINTERS

This is a good time to talk about 3D printers, which are the companion technology to 3D scans. These printers really came from the prototyping community, people who were just looking to print up small models of things they needed or were working on. They've gotten bigger and more widely used in a number of industries since they first came onto the scene, but the dental field has really taken hold of the 3D printing technology and incorporated it beautifully into the mix of digital and technological advancements used to treat patients. As noted previously, orthodontists print up models, guides, and trays for themselves and for patients. In my case, as an oral surgeon, I utilize our 3D printer to print up a real-life model which I can use as a surgical guide before I operate, allowing me to visualize and plan every step of a surgery.

3D printers have come down in cost and their accuracy has improved immensely in the past four years or so. These changes are so significant that I can count on one hand the number of orthodontists I work with who don't now use a 3D printer.

These printers are incredibly advanced, reshaping our ability to design and produce restorations of teeth that are the perfect shape and color for implant patients. There are some amazing digital libraries of teeth that provide crucial models we can use to make teeth that fit almost seamlessly with a patient's other teeth. To be fair, it's still a difficult task, even with these 3D printers, to make perfect teeth because there are so many nuances in shape and shading when it comes to teeth. But the improvement over using traditional x-ray technology is remarkable.

THE IMPORTANCE OF BEING WELL-VERSED IN DIGITAL DENTISTRY

I believe that innovation is the key to progress; if you don't learn and adapt to the latest technology, you will inevitably be surpassed. Digital dentistry is really the latest in a line of advancements the dental field has embraced. For patients, I believe it's important to seek out an oral surgeon that is, well-versed in digital dentistry. This comes from education and practice. It's important for patients to find an oral surgeon that is constantly looking for the best techniques and treatments, options that enable them to provide the very best care and thus give patients the very best results, both structurally and aesthetically.

Every patient is different, and every case is unique in some way. Digital options allow us to explore new ways to give every patient exactly the treatment they need and the outcome they want. The flexibility that digital dentistry offers lends itself to helping us give the most personalized care.

THE PATIENT ALWAYS COMES FIRST

Patient safety, comfort, and satisfaction are at the core of everything I do. Digital dentistry helps me check off all three of these things. Using the Cone Beam scanner first – which, again, gives me the most information with the least amount of radiation exposure to my patient – is the beginning of the process. Using the intraoral scans and the 3D printer makes it easy for me to thoroughly plan the course of treatment for the patient, keeping in mind that it helps me cut down the length of time I'm operating on my patient, which is safer for them and makes the recovery process easier afterward. All the digital elements I use in my practice boost my accuracy, my confidence, and that, in turn, makes the patient feel more assured and ultimately more satisfied once their case is finished.

I genuinely believe that when a patient is looking for an oral surgeon he or she should look for the doctor that has their best interest at heart and is willing to utilize every option available to give them the very best care. In my personal experience, digital dentistry plays a vital role in how effective the doctor is and the level and quality of care that he or she can offer.

DIGITAL DENTISTRY INVESTMENT

There are a number of reasons why I feel that many dentists, oral surgeons, and other doctors aren't jumping into digital dentistry. The number one concern is the expense. None of the digital options I've talked about are cheap. They are, in fact, rather expensive endeavors. I believe, from what I've seen and heard, that many doctors are afraid to make these major investments. Especially because it is new technology, and with the rapid and ever-changing advancements that occur in technology, the concern is that the technology they invest in will become outdated fairly quickly. Eventually, more money to update the technology they've invested in will be necessary. The thing to note with this is that digital dentistry is, in fact, an investment. It costs money to provide high-quality dentistry. And as with most investments, the dividends are paid out over time, with each patient, when we can offer better, safer, and more accurate care with every case we work on.

Ultimately, the upfront cost of the technology, in my opinion, more than pays for itself in two primary ways. First, we save time and money because we are able to better plan treatments and accomplish our end goal more rapidly. Second, and perhaps the more important way – at least for me – is the repayment I get when a patient sees their new smile and is overjoyed. It's not a financial repayment, but it's a big part of why I use digital dentistry.

Another reason that many practices aren't using digital dentistry is the time commitment it requires to learn to use the new technology. Whether it's a new doctor that's trying to keep their head above water and pay off loans for their new practice, or an older doctor who's been treating patients with the same techniques for his entire career, using digital dentistry takes a serious commitment to educating oneself in the various technologies and aspects of using digital guides to aid them in the treatment process. Coupled with the new advancements and the different technologies available, when a doctor decides to implement digital dentistry into their practice, it requires constantly updating oneself on the newest and latest information regarding each type of technology. This is another investment, one of time, and it's a considerable one. But in the end, the time I spent educating myself has paid for itself over and over with every case I've completed successfully.

The reality is that these concerns over digital dentistry are holding a lot of doctors and practices back from offering their patients the best care, by using the latest technology available. However, I do see that the numbers of surgeons performing guided surgeries is increasing because more and more dentists and doctors recognize the advantages. When it comes to intraoral scanners, I'd say that probably at least a quarter of oral surgeons are now using them. And when it comes to Cone Beam scanners, they are basically a standard of care at this point among oral surgeons.

THE MOUNTAIN BIKER STORY

I'd like to share one more patient story with you. Her case is another great example of how digital dentistry works in real life.

A young woman who was pregnant came to see me. She'd been mountain biking in Colorado and had a severe accident. She'd gone over the top of her handlebars, fractured her lower jaw in two places, and broke her two upper front teeth. The other four front anterior teeth were also quite loose. We were able to take Cone Beam scans before we began working to repair her jaw.

While her jaws were healing, we were able to create a digital model of her jaws and teeth, allowing us to plan how to remove the broken teeth and also where to accurately put in implants, so that we could have her temporary teeth ready right away. As soon as her jaw had healed, we placed her implants and her temporary teeth. She was able to return to work in a very short period of time, and the ultimate result she got was a beautiful smile.

A FINAL NOTE

In concluding this chapter, I feel it's important to explain a little bit about my experience with digital dentistry and why I'm passionate about staying up-to-date on the latest advancements.

I completed my oral & maxillofacial surgery residency in 2008. At that time, digital dentistry was still a new concept. There was some implant planning being done digitally. The first orthognathic cases were performed digitally shortly after that. Most of my experience with digital dentistry stems from my time in the Air Force, where I was in charge of facial traumas in Germany, working on soldiers that were coming out of Iraq and Afghanistan.

Working on these cases, employing the digital options that were available, allowed me to give my fellow soldiers the best care possible. I was able to map out a plan that would get them treated and rehabbed from their injuries as quickly as possible. The knowledge and experienced that I gained overseas was the impetus to transition into doing more digital implant dentistry when I got home.

My experience working on injured soldiers and seeing the benefits of digital dentistry in their cases, then employing those same techniques in my current practice, is what keeps me pushing to learn and utilize the latest digital and technological advancements.

At the end of the day, it all comes down to this: I want to give my patients the very best care. I want to treat each one like I treated the injured soldiers. I want each of my patients to feel safe, to feel confident, and to understand that every step of their treatment is carefully planned and that I have a backup plan as well. When their treatment is complete, seeing my patients smile, sometimes for the first time in a long time, I know that I've fulfilled my purpose. This is why I use digital dentistry, and that is why I love what I do.

About Curtis Hayes, DDS

Coal Creek Oral Surgery and Dental Implant Center
www.coalcreekoms.com

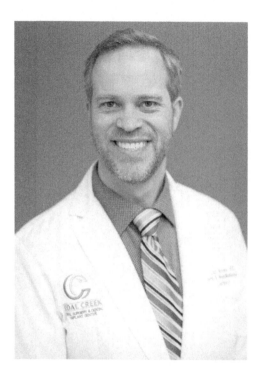

Dr. Curtis Hayes offers exceptional skill and experience to his patients seeking restorative and cosmetic dental care. A board-certified oral surgeon, Dr. Hayes completed a Bachelor of Science in Biochemistry at the United States Air Force Academy before attending the University of Colorado School of Dentistry, where he graduated *magna cum laude* in 2003.

Dr. Hayes served as a dentist at Lackland Air Force Base before continuing his education in oral surgery at Wilford Hall Medical Center in San Antonio. He also served as the Chief of Oral and Maxillofacial Surgery at Ramstein Air Force Base in Germany, where he was named 2013 US Air Force Dentist of the

Year for his care to wounded service members serving in Africa and the Middle East.

A skilled educator who has contributed to many peer-reviewed journals, Dr. Hayes has also served as the Director of Oral and Maxillofacial Surgery for the Advanced Education in General Dentistry Program. He is a member of the Colorado Society of Oral and Maxillofacial Surgeons as well as the American and Colorado Dental Associations, and is a Fellow of the American Association of Oral and Maxillofacial Surgeons and a Diplomate of the American Board of Oral and Maxillofacial Surgeons.

Dr. Hayes believes in helping to educate the public about dental care as well. He has appeared on both Colorado and National Public Radio, given interviews to the *Boulder Daily Camera*, and appeared on the USAF AOG "Checkpoints" with expert advice on opioid use in dental treatments.

Dr. Hayes has participated locally for more than twenty years as an adult leader in the Boy Scouts of America and has worked on missions to the Peruvian Amazon Basin and South Africa. He also volunteers as a clinical instructor at the University of Colorado School of Dental Medicine. Dr. Hayes and his team pride themselves on being reassuring, kind, and compassionate in addition to highly skilled.

No Fear with
Sedation Dentistry

A lot of patients experience fear and anxiety when receiving dental care or even just thinking about going to a dentist. For many patients, this fear and anxiety can be a strong enough deterrent that it prevents them from seeking care entirely or causes them to wait longer to get work done. This often means that by the time they seek help, their dental problems are very severe, and difficult and expensive to correct. The beauty of sedation dentistry is that it offers these patients security in knowing that they can be put into a much more relaxed state, enabling me and my team – or any dentist who practices sedation dentistry – to get in, treat the patient, and prevent potentially serious dental issues completely, or stop them before they reach a more critical stage.

Having a great smile is important for a patient's health and for their confidence and overall well-being in life. Sedation dentistry is another way to add to a patient's confidence and get them the dental care they want and need.

THREE BASIC TYPES OF SEDATION

When I talk with patients about sedation dentistry and putting them at ease, I think it's important for them to understand the types of sedation that are available to them, so they can get a better idea of which option might work best. I offer my input as to the method I feel would work best for them; however, the choice is always left up to the patient.

The simplest type of sedation used is nitrous oxide. Patients are fitted with a nose piece and we pump in a combination of nitrous and oxygen which relaxes them very quickly. This is also easy to reverse quickly because we're able to simply turn down the nitrous and turn up the oxygen, flooding the sedating gas from their system.

The second type of sedation is oral sedation, by means of taking a pill. After a consult, patients are given a prescription for medication to help relax them. They bring the medication with them to the dentist's office and take it before a procedure. In most cases, we prefer the patient arrives about an hour or so before the procedure and consumes the medication in the office. This technique works quite well and adds an additional level of comfort for the patient because they can administer the sedating medication to themselves, with the added benefit of knowing we're here to help them monitor its effects.

The strongest type of sedation is IV sedation. This requires an anesthesiologist. We have a dental anesthesiologist in the office for this type of sedation, someone who specializes in inserting and monitoring the IV and medication as it's administered to help keep patients calm during dental procedures.

It's important to understand that none of these methods puts a patient out completely; they generally remain conscious throughout the procedure. However, each method offers varying amounts of sedation and amnesia, with nitrous gas offering the least amount and IV sedation, of course, offering the most. We've had great success with each of these methods, and in many cases, patients remember little, if anything, about the procedure itself.

GOOD CANDIDATES FOR SEDATION DENTISTRY

Sedation dentistry is really for anyone who has high anxiety as a patient. Depending on the patient's wants and needs, the three types of sedation cover all the bases. IV sedation is typically used with the most anxious patients or for those who might be medically compromised without continuous monitoring of the sedation and how it's affecting them. Patients looking to bring themselves in and leave on their own power are the best candidates for nitrous gas. Both the oral and IV sedation techniques require the patient to bring someone with them who can drive them home.

I think it's important to point out here that good candidates for sedation dentistry are growing in number. Using sedation dentistry isn't something that should be embarrassing or make a patient feel like they are weak. For many, fear and anxiety drive them away from seeking dental services and often leads to bad experiences later on, when more aggressive treatments become necessary.

Many of the patients we see have had previous bad experiences with getting dental work done and haven't been back to a dentist for a long time. Often, their oral health is seriously compromised. Sedation dentistry is perfect for these patients because it allows them to reach a state of relaxation that makes it easier for a dentist to give them the care they need without them having to experience the fear and anxiety.

It often takes a great deal of courage for these patients to seek out the care they desperately need. For example, I saw a patient recently who hadn't been to a dentist in more than 30 years. She finally worked up the courage to be seen. It was important to let her know (and you, as the reader) that she wasn't alone. We were able to reward her courage with a relaxed visit, offering her the care she needed without causing her more physical or emotional trauma. With sedation dentistry, we are able to help remove fear and offer a pleasant experience to our patients.

MORE ABOUT A PATIENT

This seems like a good point to stop and share more about the patient I alluded to above.

The patient I'm referring to hadn't seen a dentist since 1986 and her oral health was incredibly compromised. The primary goal, of course, was to get her comfortable and then treat the most immediate problems. She had multiple areas of decay and loose teeth caused by decades of contaminant buildup that resulted in periodontal disease and other gum issues, as well as problems with her jaw bones.

We removed several teeth, just to alleviate some of the pain she experienced prior to treatment. After this visit – and more visits will inevitably be necessary – she's in much better shape than she was. She also knows that she can trust us to keep her comfortable and give her lasting results that will improve her oral health. She's less anxious now about coming back, which means I can continue to treat the issues she has and significantly improve her health.

This patient's story is a good example of why sedation dentistry works so well for people. Had the patient not been sedated, she would have been in physical and emotional distress

184

and I wouldn't have been able to accomplish as much as I did in one visit. That's part of the beauty of sedation dentistry. Many patients with backlogged dental care needs, such as this patient, prefer not to drag out the number of visits it takes to get their issues rectified. Sedation makes the patient comfortable, removes the fear of and actual feeling of pain, and allows me and my team to resolve multiple issues that we otherwise wouldn't be able to address in one visit.

For many patients, after one or two sedation appointments, trust is established and further use of sedation isn't always necessary because we've proven that we aren't going to hurt them. It's really about building trust by offering the comfort and amnesia-like qualities that sedation provides.

The other primary component of sedation dentistry is always allowing the patient to feel that they are in control of the appointment and their level of comfort. They are able to choose how much sedation they want and learn how effective it is after one visit. If they want to step down the level of sedation or remove it completely, they can. This gives them the power, which, for many, is a pleasant, new experience when it comes to dental or doctor visits.

SEDATION FOR THE NON-NERVOUS PATIENT

Sedation dentistry is still a great option even for patients who don't experience much fear or anxiety when seeing the dentist. A lot of patients, for whatever reason, need extensive dental work or a lot of different procedures that typically can only be accomplished over months and months of treatment. For these patients, appointments can sometimes seem longer when the patient is not sedated. This is largely because of the amnesia-like quality of sedation, allowing the patient to forget what's being done and how much time has passed.

Sedation is also a great tool because it can help when it's difficult to get some patients numb through local anesthetics and we have to spend a good deal of time working to get them numb and keep them numb. Fear of pain, even for patients who aren't overly nervous, is still very real and this can lead to a great deal of anxiety. In some cases, patients spend time talking to me and my staff to put off the dental work and the pain that they're afraid of. Sedation helps cut down on time in this way by putting the patient at ease, in a relaxed state, and just generally helping them get through the procedure comfortably. In the long run, sedation just helps speed the process up in general and makes it a lot more comfortable for the patient, which makes it easier for my team and me to work, which ultimately helps speed up the appointment.

"WAKING UP" AFTER SEDATION

The types of sedation we use don't really put a patient to sleep, but most patients do describe coming out of sedation as "waking up" because of the amnesiatic qualities of the medications and the fact that they are so relaxed and tend to lose track of time, much like you would after taking a nap.

As I mentioned earlier, nitrous oxide gas is the lightest form of sedation, so it is also the easiest for patients to "wake up" from. The great thing about this form of sedation is that it is easily turned on and turned off. We are simply able to turn up the nitrous to create the desired sedation. Once we've completed the work that needs to be done on the patient, we can then just as easily turn the nitrous off and turn the oxygen up, which quickly and efficiently removes the effects of the sedation. We typically allow the patient to breathe the oxygen for about 15 to 30 minutes and then they are able to go on their way under their own power.

The oral medication we use for sedation takes longer to work, which is why patients are given a prescription and have to take the tablets in advance of the appointment. In some instances, patients take the medication at home and need to have someone drive them to their appointment, as well as take them home afterward, because the effects of the sedation are longer lasting and stronger than they are with the nitrous oxide gas. We do have the patient bring the medication with them in case they need to take more to be adequately sedated. For most of our patients, they are still somewhat sedated once they leave our office and usually go home and have the best nap of their life. They usually wake up at home with little to no memory of the appointment.

IV sedation is the most drastic of all of the forms of sedation we use. It's more involved and requires, as I mentioned earlier, the presence and monitoring of an anesthesiologist. It puts patients into a much deeper state of sedation. Once the appointment is over, medication is introduced into the IV to help reverse the effects of the sedating medication. However, it's still not generally considered safe for the patient to drive, so we always insist patients have someone with them who can drive them home. Our anesthesiologist monitors the patient as they come out of the sedation, which typically takes anywhere from 30 minutes to an hour, although it may take a bit longer with some patients. It really depends on the individual patient.

SEDATION DENTISTRY ISN'T RIGHT FOR EVERYONE

It's very rare that we run into patients who can't utilize sedation for their appointments. There are, of course, issues with medication allergies that have to be considered. We also have to make sure that the patient doesn't have any underlying health issues that could make sedation risky to use. Patients with certain heart or breathing issues may not make good candidates for sedation. Also, patients with addictions to drugs or the propensity to abuse drugs aren't great candidates for sedation.

When it comes to women who are pregnant, I'm not comfortable using sedation. There are some doctors who are willing to. I tend to shy away from working on pregnant women in general, especially if they are in their first or second trimester. If they are suffering from serious oral health issues and in pain, we will, of course, work on them because the stress that pain causes is often more harmful to the child than anything we might do in an appointment. When working with women who are expecting, we always make sure to cooperate with and get a release from their OBGYN.

WHAT SEDATION DENTISTRY COSTS

As with just about any medical procedure or medication, cost varies by region, area, and doctor. For nitrous oxide gas, cost varies, however, I've rarely seen it cost more than about $100. In my office, we typically charge $30, but the final cost depends on how long the gas is needed and how much work is being done on the patient. If we end up doing a fair amount of work on a patient, we'll often waive the cost of the gas because it's so minimal in relation to the total treatment cost, but that's not something you should expect every office to do.

The cost for oral sedation is different because it's not something we can control. We write a prescription for the medication or send it to the patient's pharmacy. The cost depends a lot on if they're using insurance or a prescription medication card, or if they're paying for the medication out of pocket. I'm not an expert on drug costs and, of course, it depends on the specific medication that is used. I'd be willing to say that I can't see the prescription being more than $50, even if the patient pays out of pocket without any type of discount.

IV sedation typically starts with an initial fee, and then there are additional charges for the length of time it takes the anesthesiologist to set everything up, get the medication started, and keep the patient sedated. Again, this depends on both the doctor and the anesthesiologist. In my office, we start with an initial fee of $325 and then it costs an additional $125 for every 25-minute period of time afterward until the IV is removed.

SAVING A MARRIAGE

There's another patient story I'd like to share because I'm almost certain that sedation dentistry saved his marriage.

I had a gentleman come to see me. His wife had been on his case for years to get dental work done but his anxiety and fear kept stopping him. He was petrified. When he finally came to see me, he was in his mid-forties. He was a prominent businessman in our area, but he'd spent a great deal of time trying to hide his smile because he was embarrassed by it. His teeth were in varying degrees of deterioration and his overall smile was pretty terrible. His anterior teeth – the ones in the front – were in very bad shape.

The first time I met with him, I had to come out and sit with him in the reception area – he was too afraid to even come back to the examination area. I spoke with him for at least half an hour. I was finally able to convince him to come back for an examination, but we had to sedate him just to accomplish that. We ended up needing to rebuild his entire mouth, which is something we usually only end up doing in patients that are significantly older. His failure to smile, his pain, and his

189

embarrassment in social situations led people to believe things about him that weren't true. People often thought he was angry or upset. He was a genuinely nice, friendly man.

Once we were able to show him that using sedation would make the entire process easier and less stressful, we were able to totally transform his smile. It changed him completely. It boosted his self-confidence tremendously. Following his total mouth makeover, he'd come bebopping into our office, very sure of himself, confident in his smile, and without the overwhelming, crippling fear he'd felt when we first took his case.

COMMON CONCERNS

There are two primary concerns that most patients have when looking into sedation dentistry. Since the death of Michael Jackson and its association with Propofol – which is an incredibly strong sedating medication – patients worry about being "knocked out" and even dying. The reality is that sedation dentistry is incredibly safe when performed by skilled, educated doctors and used on patients who wouldn't be able to get the dental care they desperately need without its help.

Cost is another fairly common concern. Most of the time, patients are surprised at how inexpensive the nitrous oxide gas option and the oral medication options are. The real concern is primarily attached to IV sedation. And the reality is that it can be a pretty significant cost, depending on where it's done and how long or often it needs to be used. I try to remind patients of the fact that the few hundred dollars they spend to feel comfortable while getting the work they need done pales in comparison to the costs that could be associated with more extensive treatments they'd need down the road if they let their oral health continue to deteriorate.

ONE FINAL STORY

There's one final story I'd like to share. It paints a clear picture of why sedation dentistry plays an important role in the dentistry field and how it can help patients get their lives and their health back on track.

I was seeing a lady in her early forties who had extensive gum, bone, and tooth damage. She'd been dealing with it for years and her fear kept driving her away from seeking treatment. Eventually, as her condition continued to deteriorate, she became ever increasingly fearful of everything that would need to be done, how long it would take, and how much it would hurt. She was embarrassed that she'd let it go for so long, which was another factor that kept her away from a dentist.

When we were finally able to see her, she was sedated for her exam so we could figure out exactly what was wrong and the best courses of action. She had extensive periodontal disease and a lot of decay. There were few parts of her mouth that she could actually chew with. This had begun to impact her ability to eat and get the nutrients her body needed.

Using sedation dentistry, we did an entire oral makeover, removing teeth, treating multiple infections in her mouth, and eventually giving her a brand new smile with implants. Once the process was complete, she beamed with pride and confidence. She smiled constantly. She was able to eat and put weight on that she needed in order to feel and look healthy. Not long after we'd completed her treatment, she ended up meeting someone and getting engaged.

This woman's story is really a great example of how totally transformative sedation dentistry can be for people. At the end of the day, it's really about getting patients the care they need and a smile that they can be proud of. It's about boosting self-confidence and their overall quality of life. Sedation makes this possible by allowing patients to feel comfortable enough to come in and get the work done that they, quite often, desperately need. This is why I love sedation dentistry so much.

ABOUT J. DEREK TIEKEN, DDS

Tieken Smiles
www.TiekenSmiles.com

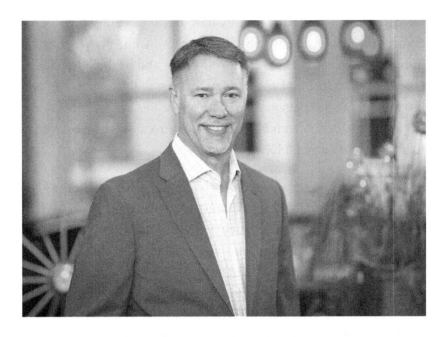

J. Derek Tieken, DDS, has spent 27 years as a dentist serving the greater Houston area and achieving numerous awards in his field.

A graduate of Baylor University and the University of Texas School of Dentistry in Houston, Dr. Tieken and his practice, Tieken Smiles Dentistry, have been recognized by many different groups for service to the community, including as "Best Dentist" by *Bay Area Houston Magazine* for 16 years in a row; one of *H-Texas Magazine's* "Top Dentists" from 2010 to 2016, and 2014 Practice of the Year by Next Level, a dental consulting and training organization. Dr. Tieken was also named a Texas Super Dentist in 2017 by *Texas Monthly*. He has also appeared on

Consumers' Research Council of America's list of top dentists in the U.S.

Dr. Tieken retains his boyhood fascination for learning about the connection between a healthy mouth and a healthy body. This dedication to consistent learning appears in his sharp focus on improving his patients' overall well-being and health. Dr. Tieken takes the time to build close relationships with his patients and provide them with personalized care as well as staying up-to-date on the latest dental trends by taking courses at The Las Vegas Institute for Advanced Dental Studies.

Dr. Tieken is a member of the American Academy of Cosmetic Dentistry and is a long-time participant in the Give Back a Smile program, which provides restorative dentistry services to victims of domestic violence and sexual assault. He also participates in many community service activities, such as giving free dental screenings to school children in the area.

Dr. Tieken and his wife of 25 years, Lori, enjoy traveling and spending time outdoors, particularly with dogs, Reese and Lacey. An avid sports enthusiast, Dr. Tieken faithfully supports Baylor University and Ole Miss, where his daughter attends school.

Dr. Tieken is strongly committed to providing Houston area patients with professional, compassionate dental service, including preventative and restorative care and TMJ treatment as well as sedation options for comfortable procedures.

AFFORDABLE COSMETIC DENTISTRY OPTIONS

According to recent statistics, 99% of the population believes that having a good smile is an important social benefit. The teeth whitening market brought in about $6 million in 2017. People value a beautiful smile because it never fails to give them confidence in their appearance and in themselves as a person. The sad fact is that many people simply cannot afford many of the expensive practices used to offer a great smile. For patients like these, they often fall into the thinking that it's all or nothing: "Either I can afford the expensive treatments, or, I just can't have a beautiful smile."

I'd like you, the reader, and all patients, to know that there are affordable cosmetic dentistry options available. You don't have to fall into the all or nothing way of thinking. In my practice alone, I'd say that a fair percentage of my patients can't afford the more expensive cosmetic options. The good news is there are a variety of different options available, including cost-friendly alternatives that enable you to pick and choose treatments based on your budget. Don't let the cost of cosmetic dentistry hold you back!

A Basic Introduction to Cosmetic Dentistry Options

I'm going to go into more detail about several different affordable cosmetic options throughout this chapter, but to start I'd like to offer just a brief overview of some of them. Many patients are under the impression that only crowns and veneers will give them the smile they're looking for. While these options are good, especially for patients with extensive damage, they are costly. There are more affordable alternatives to doing an extreme, total mouth makeover. I like to think of them as steps that lead to a smaller makeover while still giving patients the smile they're looking for.

One great option is teeth whitening. It's an affordable way to brighten up your whole mouth without being super invasive. Recontouring of teeth is another good option. In some cases, you might only need to recontour one or two teeth that stand out. Recontouring of the gum line is also an option that helps add symmetry to your smile.

Implants are another common topic in terms of correcting the appearance of a patient's smile. However, they are incredibly invasive as well as expensive. One good alternative to implants is a revolutionary device called the Snap-on Smile. It's an extremely affordable appliance that is custom fitted to a patient's teeth and, as the name indicates, simply snaps into place over a patient's existing teeth. Valpast partials are also an affordable alternative for patients with missing teeth. A great solution that is aesthetically pleasing as well. The Valplast partial is metal free, with no unsightly clasps, and looks very natural, designed to be virtually invisible in the mouth.

These are just some of the options that are available to you. My main goal here is to show you that there is more than one way to get the smile of your dreams and that it doesn't have to cost you an arm and a leg to get it!

"Fredo" the Realtor

Before I get further into the chapter, I'd like to share the story of one of my patients. His story really shows the immense impact and dramatic effects that affordable cosmetic dental procedures can have on a person's life.

Fredo, my patient, was a married realtor in his 40s. He told me that he couldn't really express himself the way he wanted to because of his smile. He constantly hid his teeth when speaking and tried hard not to reveal his teeth when he smiled, which wasn't very often. Veneers had been recommended to him by another dentist, but because they were out of his reach financially, he spent a great deal of time never knowing he could pursue affordable alternatives. When he came to my office, I discussed treatment options with him. I told him that, of course, orthodontics and veneers were ideal solutions to give him a great smile. His teeth were yellow and misaligned. He never showed his top teeth when he smiled, and his bottom teeth were especially crooked.

What I ended up suggesting to him, and ultimately giving him, was the Snap-On Smile, for both his upper and lower teeth. It was a quick, affordable option that gave him a true smile transformation. It changed his life dramatically. He started doing live videos for his business on Facebook. In all of his videos and pictures, he is smiling from ear to ear! Almost every time I see him, he tells me how this has totally changed his life. It corrected what was aesthetically displeasing about his smile, yes, but it also boosted his self-confidence and enabled him to express himself freely. It also boosted his career. By starting these videos, and by being able to carry himself confidently, he has been able to energize his career and interact better with colleagues and current and potential clients.

Fredo's story really reflects how powerful a non-invasive, quick and affordable cosmetic dental treatment can truly be.

FINDING THE RIGHT DENTIST

Just like in any other field, not all dentists are created equal. If you're interested in cosmetic procedures for your smile, you need to find the right dentist for you. Ask your friends, your family, even your coworkers, for a referral to a dentist who they've seen for a similar reason, or that has done cosmetic work on someone they know. Referrals are a really good way to find a dentist that will work with you and give you the results you're looking for. You might also want to check out dentists online, looking specifically at patient testimonials and reviews.

It's also important that you are upfront with the dentist you choose. As soon as you go into the office, make sure the staff and the dentist know exactly what you're looking for, what your financial capabilities are, and that you want to have several options to cosmetically change the look of your smile. An experienced cosmetic dentist will have patient examples – before and after photos – that they can show you.

They will also be able to tell you what options they perform, their success rate with those options, and what options they think will work best for you. Remember: you don't have to pick just one procedure. Let the dentist know you're interested in potentially doing several of the options, mixing and matching them to get the result you're looking for. An experienced dentist will help you figure out which ones will work best together to get you the smile of your dreams.

TEETH WHITENING TREATMENTS

Having white teeth is easily one of the most noticeable cosmetic aspects when it comes to your smile. Many times, someone is attending a wedding, a class reunion or a major gathering where having a white smile is a huge confidence booster, especially when talking to people they might want to impress or haven't seen in a while. A bright, white smile definitely helps when having pictures taken.

A lot of patients want to have their teeth whitened but cringe at the cost. Teeth whitening doesn't have to be expensive. In-office whitening services can run anywhere from $400 to $700, especially for the one-hour treatment. But there are lower-cost alternatives. At my practice, we offer the higher cost one hour in-office whitening which is generally the most effective. But we also offer custom take-home bleaching trays.

An impression is taken of your mouth and the bleaching tray is fabricated to fit precisely allowing the gel to be applied uniformly to all of your teeth. These range anywhere from $200 to $500. One size does not fit all. Only a small amount of gel is needed to line the tray since it fits perfectly over your existing teeth. The gel will last approximately 2 weeks and is inexpensive. If you want to touch up every now and then, you do not need to purchase a new tray, just the whitening gel and that will save money in the long run.

In comparison to the one hour in-office treatment, the take-home trays take about two to four weeks to get the best results. There are also over-the-counter whitening trays that are much less expensive. Those, however, are one-size-fits-all, which means they don't usually offer a uniformly white smile. The trays are typically worn for about an hour per day for four weeks. The cost for over-the-counter trays are usually less than $100. I don't recommend this option. Since it is a stock tray, the tray may be too big or small leading to ineffective or uneven results. But they do provide a cost-saving alternative.

The last two basic, cost-effective whitening options are whitening strips and whitening toothpaste and rinses. For young adults – from around age 13 up to about age 25 – whitening strips, I feel, are a decent option if you're on a budget. Strips usually come with 50 or 60 in a box and work very well considering how much they cost. The one negative thing to mention about strips is the fact that they can be a little difficult to keep in place, and if they slide or move, then it's difficult to achieve a uniform whitening of your teeth. Also, unlike custom trays which can be reused, whitening strips are not reusable so there is an expense if buying more.

When it comes to whitening toothpastes and rinses, you get what you pay for. These options only remove surface stains. If you've had in-office whitening procedures, or have used strips or trays, whitening toothpaste or rinses are a good thing to add to your daily regimen.

For the best value, I would recommend either the one hour in-office treatment or the take-home trays. These offer the best results and aren't as expensive as some other cosmetic procedures might be. Please consult your dentist before doing any type of whitening treatment, especially if you are considering over-the-counter and take home products. Please note, if you have crowns or tooth colored restorations on the teeth you're whitening, they won't change color. Your teeth will get lighter, but the crowns and restorations will remain the same. Ultimately, the money spent to get a uniformly white smile will be wasted and the results will be uneven. The solution to this is easy. Whiten your teeth first, then replace the crowns and composite fillings. Regardless of which option you choose to go with, consult your dentist and follow their advice.

RECONTOURING

Tooth recontouring or tooth reshaping is one of the most convenient, cost-effective options for fixing chipped, uneven or poorly aligned teeth to create a more attractive smile. Because it is relatively inexpensive and non-invasive, it is a good place to start. This type of treatment is perfect for patients that may have some type of shape irregularity with their teeth. This irregularity might just be the tooth shape they were born with. In other cases, they might have sustained cracks, chips, or other types of damage to their teeth. Recontouring is also aesthetically helpful when a patient has some teeth that are significantly longer than others. If minor cosmetic dental problems make you afraid to smile, cosmetic contouring may be right for you.

Small amounts of tooth enamel are removed to change a tooth's length, surface, or overall shape. This improves the look of a patient's smile by balancing out the way your smile looks, creating a more harmonious-looking smile plane. In the grand scheme of cosmetic procedures, recontouring is one of the most conservative. It can generally be done in one visit, involves a minimum amount of discomfort – if any, no anesthesia is required and the results are immediately visible.

To give you a better understanding of what the recontouring procedure is, let me explain it step by step. When a patient comes in to have their teeth reshaped, the dentist utilizes a tool with a sandpaper disc or a fine diamond bur to remove very small portions of a tooth's enamel.

Sandpaper discs are especially helpful when trying to reach imperfections in-between two teeth. The entire area that's been recontoured is then polished and buffed to make sure the tooth is smooth to prevent any tearing or rubbing inside the patient's mouth. All of this is done without ever touching the nerve of the tooth, which sits much deeper, past the enamel. Again, no anesthesia or novocaine (numbing medication) is needed for this procedure. If the tooth's enamel layer is too thin or if the pulp lies too close to the tooth's surface, recontouring may not be possible and another procedure, such as bonding or veneers, might need to be considered instead.

Keep in mind that once removed, enamel can't be replaced. This means that it's important to find a skilled dentist that you trust to perform this procedure. The goal is to remove the absolute least amount of enamel necessary while getting the desired aesthetic result.

As I mentioned, recontouring results are immediate. The results depend entirely on how much the imperfections stand out. For patients with a lot of damage to their teeth, recontouring can dramatically improve the continuity and flow of their teeth and therefore of their smile. No follow up treatments are necessary after the treatment is complete.

This procedure can reshape extremely long teeth or extremely pointed teeth to make them look more round and smooth. Ultimately, the results are going to be most noticeable to the patient who's lived with, and been affected by, how their smile looks to them. At the end of the day, even if you are the only one who really notices a big change, it will boost your confidence in your smile and in yourself. A change in the way you carry yourself might sometimes be the most noticeable change of all. And that's true for just about any cosmetic procedure.

CROWNS

As I mentioned at the beginning of this chapter, when it comes to cosmetic procedures, it doesn't have to be all or nothing. Using crowns to correct aesthetic smile issues becomes expensive if you place one on every tooth with an imperfection. They can be very cost-effective, however, when used sparingly.

Placing a single crown on a front tooth is one of the most challenging procedures a dentist can face. It is incredibly difficult to place, fit, and match one crown to the rest of the patient's teeth. A crown in the front of your mouth is, of course, extremely noticeable, so it's important to find a dentist that is skilled at placing crowns and who also works closely with a trained, experienced dental lab that can create a beautiful, well-matched crown.

In my opinion, it's best to go with an all porcelain/ceramic crown because it is more translucent and therefore looks more natural. All ceramic crowns give patients and dentists the best of both worlds. They are strong and aesthetic! Using ceramic crowns also means that the patient won't have any black or dark areas showing around the gum line. This can happen if a metal-based crown is used, even if porcelain is placed on top.

That's why we only use all-porcelain/ceramic in my office. I favor E-max brand porcelain crowns. At this time, E-max is the material of choice by most cosmetic dentists and laboratories. This material allows the crown to be bonded to your tooth, giving a much tighter fit at the margins. They are one of the strongest brands, which is important for the overall structure of a patient's bite and which means that they are less likely to break or wear down. E-max crowns are also my personal favorite in terms of aesthetics.

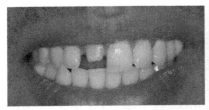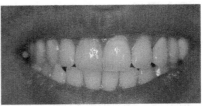

Placing a single crown

Remember, it's important to consult with a dentist before seeking this treatment option. Some dentists, while good at placing multiple crowns, aren't as experienced when it comes to placing single crowns. In order to get the best results possible, you want to find a dentist who is specifically experienced in the exact type of treatment that you are requesting.

When placing crowns on back molars, I recommend zirconia crowns which are unbreakable! This will save the patient money in the long run as zirconia crowns are very durable.

BONDING

Bonding is another great, affordable cosmetic option for individuals who have cracked, chipped, or damaged teeth. Basically, this procedure gets its name from the fact that a high-intensity curing light and an adhesive are used with tooth-colored resin materials which are bonded to the teeth to fill in any imperfections. Bonding can also be used to improve the appearance of discolored teeth, to lengthen teeth, to close spaces or gaps between teeth, and to entirely change the shape of teeth. Veneers are often used to fix some of these issues, but veneers aren't always a financial option for everyone. Bonding is significantly less expensive.

As well as being cost-effective, bonding is also an incredibly simple procedure to do. Still, as with the majority of the procedures mentioned in this chapter – and, really, with ANY procedure – it's vital to use a skilled cosmetic dentist. This is because it is particularly difficult to match a bond versus a veneer. And although bonding requires just one visit, it also is more likely to stain and is less natural looking than a veneer. Still, the fact is that bonding is fast, painless, and is one of the most commonly used and affordable treatments.

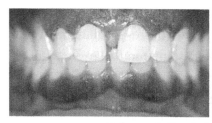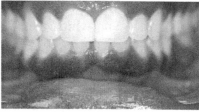

Before and after closing gaps with bonding

Bonding isn't as strong as your natural teeth, so the use of this option requires you to be more careful when doing things like eating or sports activities. The fee varies from approximately $150 to $850 per tooth for bonding versus 1000-2200 per tooth for veneers. Of course, costs of dental bonding depend on your specific dental conditions, amount of teeth that need cosmetic repair, and the dentist performing the operation. Overall, bonding is another great, affordable cosmetic treatment.

A FEW WELL-PLACED VENEERS

I've mentioned the costliness of veneers several times already throughout this chapter. What I want people to understand is that while veneers are definitely one of the costlier cosmetic options, they can still be on the table without breaking the bank. The key is to have a few, critically-placed veneers to give you the most bang for your buck, possibly in combination with other procedures such as whitening.

To be completely honest, veneers are the "best it gets" when it comes to cosmetic dental procedures. They offer outstanding cosmetic results and are very strong and long-lasting. But to get a mouthful of them would set you back tens of thousands of dollars. Instead, it's more cost effective to consult with your dentist to explain the specific parts of your smile that are bothering you.

Together, you can determine how your smile can best be transformed and which teeth to focus on to get the end results you're looking for. In most cases, something like eight to ten veneers is recommended. But, depending on what you need to get the smile you're looking for, I might be able to put in just two or four veneers in the right places and still manage to create your dream smile.

CONFIDENCE FOR ELIZABETH

I'd like to share another story here, one that beautifully illustrates the power of a few well-placed veneers.

Elizabeth was a lovely patient of mine in her 50s. Four of her front teeth were chipped really badly. Ultimately, she wanted to do a total smile makeover. She'd lost confidence in herself and was embarrassed by the way her smile looked. She'd been trying to put herself back out into the dating world, but because of her teeth, she didn't feel confident enough to get started on some of the online dating websites available. When she came to my office, I was able to give her four beautiful veneers, strategically placed to cover up the teeth that had the most damage and that were the most noticeable when she smiled. By fixing these few flaws, it gave her a smile that she was confident to show off. She ended up getting back out there, and today, she's happily involved in a relationship.

Elizabeth's story, while simple, is a good example of how easily someone's life can be transformed with minimal, affordable cosmetic dentistry.

GUM RECONTOURING

Another issue that poses smile problems for some patients is asymmetry with their gums. Veneers are also often used to fix this, however, because veneers are so pricey, gum recontouring is a good alternative. Basically, we reshape the gum tissue around your teeth to make it as symmetrical – and aesthetically pleasing – as possible, while making sure it still looks natural. Asymmetrical gums often make a person's teeth look misaligned, or make one tooth look longer or shorter than another. Evening up the gums makes a person's teeth and smile look proportionate and natural.

Gum recontouring involves removal of some gum tissue and does require a local anesthetic, but it's still a fairly simple procedure that can usually be done in one short visit. A soft tissue laser is used to trim away and recontour the excess gum at the gum line. This procedure usually doesn't involve a significant amount of discomfort, and because a laser is used, there's no bleeding and no need for stitches.

I treated a young woman once, a dental student in fact, who had excess gum over two of her front teeth. She was getting ready to graduate and wanted to celebrate, but she was unhappy with the way her smile looked because of her gums. We were able to recontour her gums around her front teeth. She was absolutely thrilled with how things turned out. As a soon-to-be dentist, she seemed to want to practice what she would be preaching. By getting her smile fixed, she was more confident to go out and take on the world of dentistry.

THE SNAP-ON SMILE

The Snap-On Smile that I talked about earlier is my favorite affordable procedure. For the last seven years or so, the Snap-On Smile has been quickly and affordably transforming peoples' smiles. It's an appliance made out of a patented hi-tech acetyl resin that snaps over your existing teeth. It is completely removable, requires no adhesives, alters no tooth structure, does not stain and you can eat and drink with it! Only two appointments are needed, the first to take an impression and the second to deliver the appliance. You must be evaluated by a dentist to make sure your teeth and gums are healthy and you are a good candidate.

Ultimately, the Snap-On Smile is perfect for people who dislike the shape and/or color of their smile. This appliance can be used to replace missing teeth, as a cosmetic enhancement, open the bite or as a temporary while undergoing dental implants. The Snap-On Smile gives them a temporary set of teeth to use until the implants are placed.

Snap-On Smile is life changing! I have done literally hundreds and it is available for upper and lower teeth. It's easy to care for and can be a temporary or long-term provisional cosmetic solution.

Snap-On Smile ranges between $1,500 and $2500 per appliance. But it's important to note that they're completely customized using digital impressions of the patient's existing teeth, ultimately allowing the appliance to easily snap right into place. The entire mouth is transformed literally with a snap. Other treatments such as veneers and braces can be very expensive.

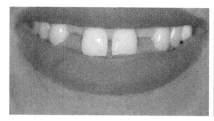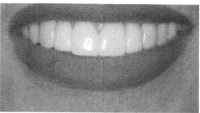

Snap on Smile - Before and After

The Snap-On Smile is a relatively new addition to affordable cosmetic dentistry so not every dentist may offer it. I've been working with this appliance for a long time and I'm well-versed in using it. So much so, that I lecture throughout the country to other dentists interested in adding the Snap-On Smile as a treatment option for their patients. It's important to make sure that if you're looking at the Snap-On Smile as an option, you find a dentist who has worked with it extensively and offers it routinely in their practice.

MY MOTTO, MY PASSION

I have this saying, a motto of sorts: "A beautiful smile speaks when you don't." It's my own little trademark. Honestly, I don't think you have to have a "perfect" smile, just one that is pleasing. Most important of all, it needs to be a smile that you're proud of and confident in. At the end of the day, I just want to give all of my patients a smile that boosts confidence.

Also, I want everyone thinking about cosmetic dentistry to understand that they don't have to fall into the all or nothing way of thinking. There are many available cosmetic dental procedures out there, many of which are affordable and can be mixed and matched with one another to give you the very best results at a reasonable price. I want to give you a smile that speaks for you when you don't. I want that same smile to communicate confidence and beauty, on the outside as well as on the inside. That's why I love my job. And that's why I do what I do.

ABOUT TERRI ALANI, DDS

Terri Alani, DDS
www.TexasToothLady.com

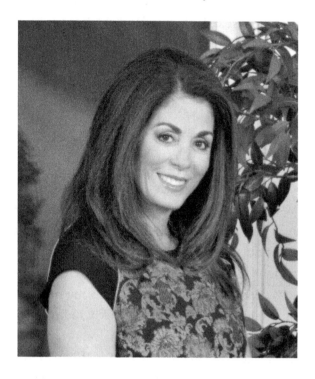

Dr. Terri Alani, a former Texas Aggie, has spent the past 30 years creating a successful practice in Houston one smile at a time.

Dr. Alani graduated from Texas A&M University with a Bachelor of Science degree, then went on to attend the University of Texas Houston dental school, where she graduated with a DDS.

Dr. Alani's motto, "A beautiful smile speaks when you don't," has become a guiding principle in her practice. Along with her priority on patient care, her attention to creating beautiful smiles has led to a multitude of referrals.

Cosmetic dentistry is Dr. Alani's focus, but her office incorporates all phases of general dentistry from teeth cleaning to smile makeovers. She incorporates her passion for fitness, including swimming, skiing, and weight training, into her practice. Her enthusiasm for good health leads her to be pro-active in patient care. Dr. Alani conducts routine check-ups so patients remain in good health.

Dr. Alani lectures nationally to dentists teaching the Snap-On-Smile procedure. She is also a monthly guest on "Great Day Houston" with Debra Duncan where she discusses dental-related topics. She is the Media Committee Chairman for the Greater Houston District Dental Society and serves on the Communications Committee for the Texas Dental Association. For the past 8 years, she has been voted as one of Houston's Top Dentists. Dr. Alani has also hosted a weekly radio show for seven years with her brother, Dr. Wayne Alani, an orthopedic surgeon. They now have a television medical show "What's Up Doc?" Her YouTube channel which was started in 2017 now has over 13,000 subscribers. She has been involved in community outreach programs to help the underprivileged receive dental care as well as the oral cancer awareness walk in Houston.

Dr. Alani is a member of the Greater Houston Dental Society, Texas Dental Association, American Dental Association and is on the Advisory Council for the College of Science at Texas A&M.